RELATIONSHIPS IN DERMATOLOGY

Other titles in the *New Clinical Applications* Series:

Dermatology (Series Editor Dr J. L. Verbov)
Dermatological Surgery
Superficial Fungal Infections
Talking Points in Dermatology – I
Treatment in Dermatology
Current Concepts in Contact Dermatitis
Talking Points in Dermatology – II
Tumours, Lymphomas and Selected Paraproteinaemias

Cardiology (Series Editor Dr D. Longmore)
Cardiology Screening

Rheumatology (Series Editors Dr J. J. Calabro and Dr W. Carson Dick)
Ankylosing Spondylitis
Infections and Arthritis

Nephrology (Series Editor Dr G. R. D. Catto)
Continuous Ambulatory Peritoneal Dialysis
Management of Renal Hypertension
Chronic Renal Failure
Calculus Disease
Pregnancy and Renal Disorders
Multisystem Diseases
Glomerulonephritis I
Glomerulonephritis II

NEW
CLINICAL
APPLICATIONS
DERMATOLOGY

RELATIONSHIPS IN DERMATOLOGY

Editor

JULIAN L. VERBOV
JP, MD, FRCP, FIBiol

Consultant Dermatologist
Royal Liverpool Hospital,
Liverpool, UK

KLUWER ACADEMIC PUBLISHERS
DORDRECHT / BOSTON / LONDON

Distributors

for the United States and Canada: Kluwer Academic Publishers, PO Box 358, Accord Station, Hingham, MA 02018-0358, USA
for all other countries: Kluwer Academic Publishers Group, Distribution Center, PO Box 322, 3300 AH Dordrecht, The Netherlands

British Library Cataloguing in Publication Data

Relationships in dermatology.
1. Medicine. Dermatology
I. Verbov, Julian II. Series
616.5

ISBN-13: 978-94-010-7686-9 e-ISBN-13: 978-94-009-2629-5
DOI: 10.1007/978-94-009-2629-5

Published in the United Kingdom by Kluwer Academic Publishers, PO Box 55, Lancaster, UK.

Kluwer Academic Publishers BV incorporates the publishing programmes of D. Reidel, Martinus Nijhoff, Dr W. Junk and MTP Press.

CONTENTS

LIST OF AUTHORS

Professor G. H. Elder, BA, MD, FRCPath MRCP
Professor of Medical Biochemistry,
University of Wales College of Medicine and
Honorary Consultant in Chemical Pathology,
South Glamorgan Health Authority,
Heath Park,
Cardiff CF4 4XN

Dr S. R. Porter, BSc, BDS, PhD, FDSRCS
Hon. Lecturer in Oral Medicine and Oral Surgery,
University Dept of Oral Medicine, Surgery and Pathology,
Bristol Dental School and Hospital,
Lower Maudlin Street,
Bristol BS1 2LY

Dr C. M. E. Rowland Payne, MB, MRCP
Lecturer and Hon. Senior Registrar in Dermatology,
Westminster Hospital,
University of London,
London SW1

Professor C. Scully, BSc, BDS, MBBS, PhD, FDSRCPS, MRCPath.
Professor of Oral Medicine and Oral Surgery,
University Dept of Oral Medicine, Surgery and Pathology,
Bristol Dental School and Hospital,
Lower Maudlin Street,
Bristol BS1 2LY

Mr P. Wright, FRCS, DO
Consultant Ophthalmic Surgeon,
Moorfields Eye Hospital,
City Road,
London EC1V 2PD

SERIES EDITOR'S FOREWORD

This is the eighth volume in the *New Clinical Applications Dermatology* Series. Awareness of relationships is of prime importance in dermatology. Professor Scully and Dr Porter cover the skin and mouth in a comprehensive and informative manner. Mr Peter Wright effortlessly and concisely brings the eye and the skin together. Dr C. Rowland Payne both relates and speculates on the enigma of sarcoidosis. Professor Elder concludes the book with a scholarly update on porphyria and the skin.

I thank all the above for their fine contributions. This volume should have widespread appeal.

JULIAN VERBOV

ABOUT THE EDITOR

Dr Julian Verbov is Consultant Dermatologist to Liverpool Health Authority and Honorary Clinical Lecturer in Dermatology at the University of Liverpool.

He is a member of the British Association of Dermatologists, representing the British Society for Paediatric Dermatology on its Executive Committee. He is Editor of the Proceedings of the North of England Dermatological Society. He is a Fellow of the Zoological Society of London and a Member of the Society of Authors. He is a popular national and international speaker and author of more than 200 publications.

His special interests include paediatric dermatology, inherited disorders, dermatoglyphics, pruritus ani, cutaneous polyarteritis nodosa, therapeutics, drug abuse and medical humour. He organizes the British Postgraduate Course in Paediatric Dermatology and is a Member of the Editorial Board of *Clinical and Experimental Dermatology*.

1

THE MOUTH AND THE SKIN

C. SCULLY AND S. R. PORTER

The oral mucosa is similar in structure to skin, consisting of stratified squamous epithelium, but it lacks a stratum lucidum and appendages such as hair and apocrine glands. Essentially protective in nature, the oral mucosa is extremely sensitive, more so than most areas of skin, and in certain regions contains taste buds, in others minor salivary glands.

However, despite their clear structural and functional similarities, the skin and oral mucosa vary in disease susceptibility; the reasons for this remain in large part unexplained. There are also considerable variations in the structure and disease susceptibility of the oral mucosa in different sites of the mouth. The oral mucosa is conventionally divided into masticatory, lining and specialized types, and it is the masticatory mucosa which, in general, is less prone to manifest mucosal diseases.

There are interesting associations in disease susceptibility between oral and cutaneous tissues. For example, the teeth, which are ectodermal derivatives, may be affected in some ectodermoses (such as ectodermal dysplasia) and there are associations between dental and nail defects (such as in chronic mucocutaneous candidosis). Similarities between mucosal and skin responses are shown, for example, by the association of hypertrichosis with both congenital and the various forms of drug-induced gingival hyperplasia.

THE NORMAL MOUTH AND BENIGN VARIANTS

Diagnostic confusion is not infrequently caused by benign conditions such as sebaceous glands in the lips or buccal mucosa (Fordyce spots; Figure 1.1); leukoedema (a filmy opalescence of the buccal mucosa); racial pigmentation; foliate papillae on the tongue; a hairy tongue and geographic tongue.

Geographic tongue (erythema migrans; benign migratory glossitis) is a benign condition of unknown aetiology found in up to 2% of patients. A higher prevalence is found in patients with a fissured (scrotal) tongue, and in psoriasis; a similar lesion may be found in Reiter's syndrome. Geographic tongue may be asymptomatic or may cause mild soreness. Irregular pink or red depapillated areas are often circumscribed by a raised yellowish border. The lesions change in size, shape and site over hours to days. No treatment is required.

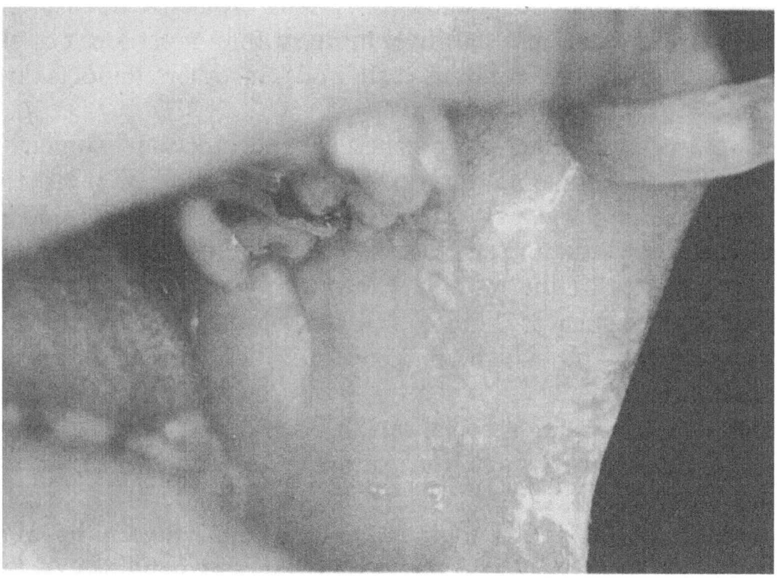

FIGURE 1.1 Fordyce spots

DISEASE RELATIONSHIPS

Some diseases affect either mouth or skin or both oral mucosa and skin. A range of systemic disorders can produce oral and/or skin lesions (Tables 1.1 and 1.2).

Oral lesions are important since they may:

(a) Be an early or even presenting feature of the disease;
(b) Be an essential diagnostic feature;
(c) Produce the most important symptoms as far as the patient is concerned;
(d) Predispose to other complications.

Clinical diagnosis of oral lesions should be somewhat easier than dermatological clinical diagnosis, since a more restricted range of local and systemic diseases appear to manifest in the mouth. In fact, oral diagnosis can be more difficult for the physician who has had little training in oral diagnosis, especially in view of the more dynamic state of oral than skins lesions. Many oral lesions break down and ulcerate because they are exposed to moisture, infection and trauma. Indeed ulcers are the most common oral mucosal lesions and can have a very varied aetiology (Table 1.3). The history is therefore of paramount importance in oral diagnosis and special investigations, especially biopsy, are often warranted. However, although theoretically little more difficult than skin biopsy, an oral biopsy is probably a less pleasant or acceptable procedure for the patient and is, without special care, more likely to damage the normal anatomy (such as the parotid duct) or to leave after-pain and swelling. Furthermore, it is important in the diagnosis of epithelial disorders to biopsy perilesional tissue and not simply an ulcer (which has virtually no epithelium!), and also to avoid areas with unrelated pathology (such as gingiva inflamed because of bacterial plaque accumulation). A further complicating factor in diagnosis is that oral lesions sometimes show histopathological changes at variance with skin lesions; oral lichen planus, for example, not infrequently lacks the saw-toothing of epithelial rete ridges.

Since it is impossible to discuss all aspects of the mouth–skin relationship, this review is restricted to:

(a) Skin diseases that often affect the mouth;

TABLE 1.1 Oral manifestations in some diseases with common skin manifestations

Disease	*Oral manifestations*
Acanthosis nigricans	White papilliferous lesions, fissured tongue and lips
Addison's disease	Pigmentation
Amyloidosis	Bullae, purpura, macroglossia, mucosal fibrosis and calcification
Behçet's syndrome	Ulcers
Bloom syndrome	Cheilitis
Chickenpox	Ulcers
Dermatomyositis	Telangiectasia, oedema, white lesions
Hand, foot and mouth disease	Ulcers
Kawasaki's disease (mucocutaneous lymph node syndrome)	Sore tongue, cheilitis
Lupus erythematosus	White lesions, ulcers, Sjögren's syndrome
McCune–Albright syndrome	Enlargement of the maxilla and mandible
Measles	Koplik's spots
Papillomavirus infections	Verruca vulgaris, condylomata acuminatum, papillomas
Pityriasis rosea	Red macules
Polyarteritis nodosa	Ulcers, nodules, papules, erythema
Porphyria (erythropoietic)	Red discoloured teeth
Reiter's syndrome	Ulcers or red raised lesions
Sarcoidosis	Salivary gland swelling Xerostomia Lumps in mouth
Scleroderma	Stiffness of lips and tongue, trismus, telangiectasia, periodontal ligament widening, Sjögren's syndrome
Zoster	Pain and ulcers in mandibular or maxillary zoster

TABLE 1.2 Oral manifestations of genetically determined diseases involving the skin and appendages or mucosae

Disease	*Oral manifestations*
Acanthosis nigricans (benign type)	Verrucous plaques
Acrodermatitis enteropathica (Danbolt–Closs syndrome)	Ulcers, perioral pustular eruptions
Chondroectodermal dysplasia (Ellis–van Creveld syndrome)	Hypodontia, dental anomalies, midline defect in upper lip
Cowden syndrome (multiple hamartoma and neoplasia syndrome)	Papillomatous lesions
Darier–White disease	White lesions
Dyskeratosis congenita (Zinsser–Engmann–Cole syndrome)	Blisters, white lesions
Ectodermal dysplasia	Hypodontia, dental anomalies, delayed eruption
Ehlers–Danlos syndrome	Severe periodontitis, dental anomalies, hypermobility of the tongue, increased mucosal fragility, TMJ dislocation
Epidermolysis bullosa	Dental hypoplasia, plaque-associated diseases, blisters, erosions and scarring
Fabry syndrome	(Rarely) telangiectasia
Gardner's syndrome	Osteomas, unerupted teeth
Goltz syndrome (focal dermal hypoplasia)	Papillomatosis, cleft lip/palate Dental abnormalities (e.g. hypodontia, delayed eruption)
Gorlin–Goltz syndrome (multiple basal cell naevi syndrome)	Odontogenic keratocysts
Hereditary benign intraepithelial dyskeratosis	White lesions
Hereditary haemorrhagic telangiectasia	Telangiectasia
Hyalinosis cutis et mucosae (lipoid proteinosis. Urbach–Wiethe syndrome)	Immobile tongue Waxy plaques, immobile tongue, ulcers, dental abnormalities
Incontinentia pigmenti (Bloch–Sulzberger syndrome)	Hypodontia or hyperdontia Hypoplastic teeth, delayed eruption
Pachyonychia congenita (Jadassohn–Lewandowski syndrome)	Thickened white oral mucosa

Disease	*Oral manifestations*
Maffucci syndrome	Haemangiomas
Neurofibromatosis	Neurofibromas
Papillon–Lefevre syndrome	Severe periodontitis
Peutz–Jeghers syndrome	Melanosis
Pityriasis rubra pilaris	White lesions
Porokeratosis (Mibelli's disease)	Atrophic lesions with white borders
Pseudoxanthoma elasticum (Grönblad–Strandberg syndrome)	Intramucosal nodules
Sjögren–Larsson syndrome	Hypoplastic teeth
Sturge–Weber syndrome	Angioma, complications of phenytoin
Tuberous sclerosis	Enamel pits, fibrous lesions
Tylosis	Leukoplakia
White sponge naevus	White folded mucosa
Xanthomatosis	Xanthomas
Xeroderma pigmentosum	(Rarely) carcinoma

(b) Less common subepithelial vesiculobullous disorders;
(c) Skin diseases in which oral lesions significantly contribute to diagnosis;
(d) Diseases involving the mouth–skin interface (the lips).

SKIN DISEASES THAT OFTEN AFFECT THE MOUTH

No skin diseases commonly have oral manifestations, but oral lichen planus is relatively common. Mucous membrane pemphigoid and oral erythema multiforme are the only other dermatoses seen with any frequency in a dental clinic.

Lichen planus (LP)

Oral lichen planus affects up to 2% of the population. It is often asymptomatic, but patients may note white lesions or complain of

TABLE 1.3 Causes of oral ulceration

Local causes	Systemic Disease
Trauma	(a) *Cutaneous disease*
Chemical	Lichen planus
Physical	Pemphigus
Thermal	Pemphigoid
Radiation	Erythema multiforme
Artefactual	Dermatitis herpetiformis
Neoplastic causes	Linear IgA disease
Carcinoma	Epidermolysis bullosa
Salivary neoplasms	(b) *Connective tissue disease*
Melanoma	Lupus erythematosus
Lymphoma	Felty's syndrome
Others	Reiter's syndrome
Aphthae	(c) *Haematological disease*
Recurrent aphthae and Behcet's syndrome	Anaemia or deficiency states
	Leukopenia
	Leukaemia
	(d) *Gastrointestinal*
	Crohn's disease
	Coeliac disease
	Ulcerative colitis
	(e) *Infections*
	Herpesviruses
	Coxsackie viruses
	HIV
	Acute ulcerative gingivitis
	Mycobacterial infections
	Syphilis
	Histoplasmosis/blastomycosis
	(f) *Drugs*
	Cytotoxic agents
	Phenytoin
	Others

oral soreness or dryness. Two thirds of patients are females; most are of late middle age. Up to 70% of patients presenting with cutaneous LP have oral LP; conversely, less than 30% of patients presenting with oral LP have cutaneous involvement. Oral lesions affect mainly the buccal mucosa, less commonly the tongue or gums, and rarely the palate. Oral LP is almost invariably bilateral and, unlike cutaneous LP, is remarkably persistent – for even as long as 25 years or more[1].

A typical patient with lichen planus, therefore, is a middle-aged female complaining of persistent soreness in both buccal mucosae.

Clinical appearance

The most common clinical appearance of oral LP is a network of white lines (Wickham's striae) in the buccal mucosa, bilaterally and posteriorly (reticular lichen planus: Figure 1.2). White papules, plaques resembling leukoplakia, atrophic areas and erosions are less common. Bullous LP is *exceedingly* rare. Different clinical forms may

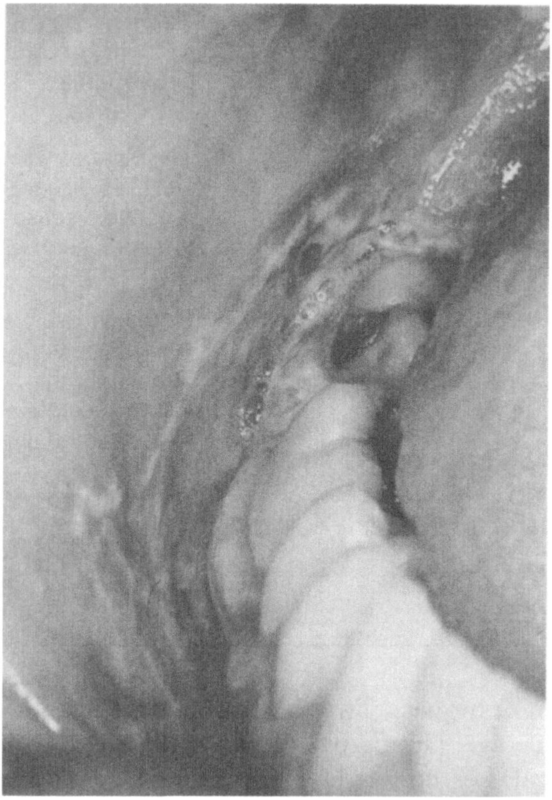

FIGURE 1.2 Reticular pattern of oral lichen planus

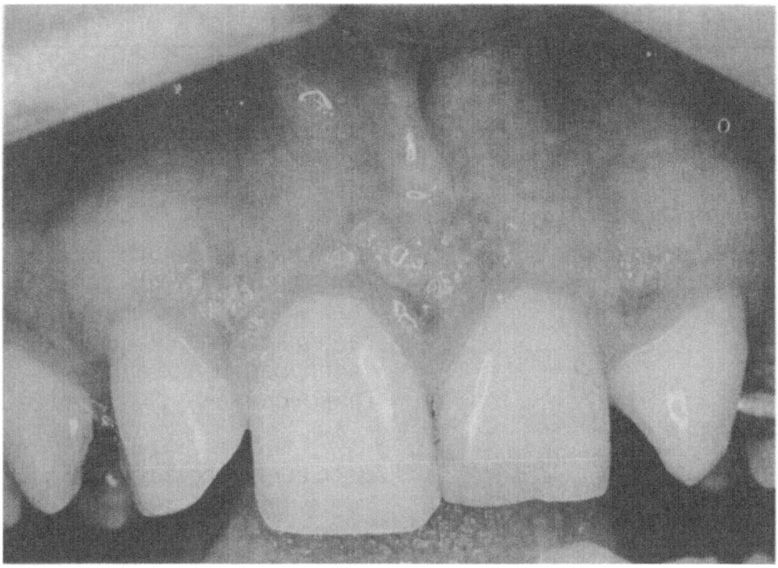

FIGURE 1.3 Desquamative gingivitis – this can be an oral manifestation of lichen planus or mucous membrane pemphigoid

be intermixed in a single patient, or there may be change from one form to another. Smoking appears to predispose to plaque-type lesions in LP-affected patients.

Gingival involvement may cause white lesions and/or desquamative gingivitis (Figure 1.3).

Prognosis

Oral LP is often persistent but is usually benign. There is about a 1% chance of malignant transformation over 5 years, and this occurs predominantly in those with long-standing erosive LP. Atrophic LP clinically closely resembles erythroplasia – a premalignant condition.

Aetiology

The factors predisposing to oral LP are unclear and the evidence suggests a much lower prevalence of systemic disease, such as liver

TABLE 1.4 Proposed aetiologies and associations in oral lichen planus

Infection	
Bacteria	No evidence
Viruses	Not completely excluded
Psychogenic	
Stress	No evidence
Drugs/Chemicals	
Dental restorations	Not completely excluded
Drugs	Lichenoid lesions with non-steroidal anti-inflammatory agents; antimalarials; antidiabetics; antihypertensives and antimicrobials
Miscellaneous	
Rheumatoid arthritis Diabetes Hypertension	Associations occasionally ? related to drug therapy
Immunological Disorders	
Graft versus host disease (GVHD)	Lichenoid lesions in GVHD
Lupus erythematosus	Rare overlap syndromes
Liver disease	No association with oral LP proven

disease, than has appeared in some reports of cutaneous LP (Table 1.4). Suggested associations of oral LP with systemic disease such as diabetes mellitus and hypertension (Grinspan syndrome) are most probably explained by drug-induced lichenoid lesions[1].

Diagnosis

The history and clinical appearance are usually highly indicative of the diagnosis of oral LP when white lesions are obvious, but lesional biopsy is often indicated, usually to exclude:

(a) lupus erythematosus
(b) leukoplakia (keratosis)
(c) malignancy

Histology in oral LP may show hyperkeratosis, acanthosis, basal cell liquefaction, Civatte bodies, and a dense mononuclear cell infiltrate in the lamina propria, but a saw-tooth configuration of the rete pegs is not common.

Management

Symptomatic oral LP may respond to topical corticosteroids (Table 1.5). Recalcitrant lesions can be managed with intralesional corticosteroids and rarely vitamin A derivatives (such as etretinate), dapsone or immunosuppressive agents.

TABLE 1.5 Management of oral lichen planus

Hydrocortisone sodium succinate	2.5 mg pellets q.i.d.
Triamcinolone acetonide	In orabase – applied q.i.d.
Betamethasone sodium phosphate	Two 0.5 mg tablets dissolved in 15 ml mouthwash (not swallowed), used q.i.d.
Betamethasone valerate	100 μg of spray, used q.i.d.

Mucous membrane pemphigoid (MMP)

Oral mucous membrane pemphigoid is less common than LP but usually symptomatic, patients complaining of oral blisters, ulcers or soreness. Oral lesions occur in most patients and usually precede lesions elsewhere. Most patients are females in their late middle age. Other mucosal surfaces can be involved (e.g. conjunctivae, vagina), but often oral lesions are the only complaint. Any site in the mouth can be affected, but rarely the hard palate[2,3].

Clinical appearance

Intact vesicles or blisters may be seen and the Nikolsky sign can be positive. Blisters may break down to leave irregular fibrin-covered superficial erosions (Figure 1.4). Healing may be associated with scarring. MMP may (like LP) produce a desquamative gingivitis.

Prognosis

The oral lesions of MMP are benign but persistent. Oral MMP has a weak association with internal malignancy.

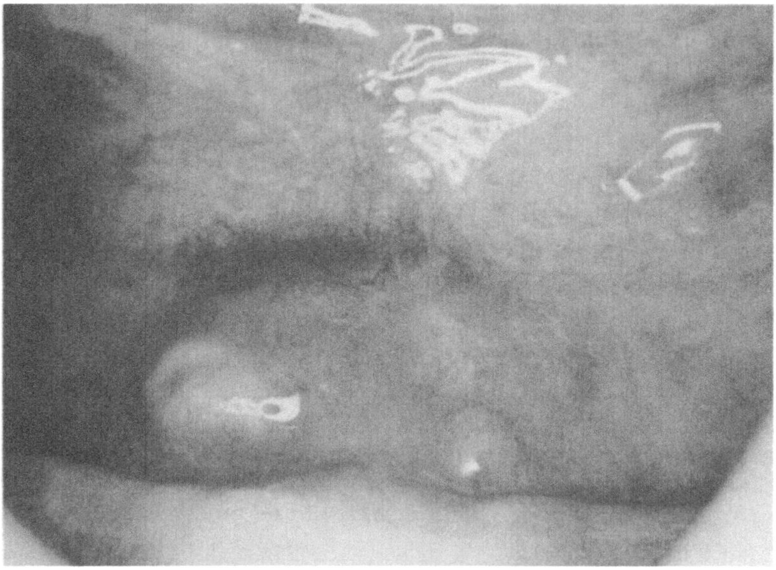

FIGURE 1.4 Mucous membrane pemphigoid of the palate

Aetiology

The aetiology of oral MMP is unclear but may be autoimmune. Rare cases are drug-induced (e.g. by frusemide or penicillamine). Some patients have a non-immunologically based but clinically similar disease presenting with blood blisters often restricted to the oral mucosa alone (angina bullosa haemorrhagica)[4].

Diagnosis

The history and clinical appearances are often suggestive of MMP but cannot reliably differentiate from pemphigus or, indeed, from other vesiculobullous disorders (Table 1.3). Biopsy (including immunostaining) is therefore essential and shows subepithelial vesiculation with deposits of C3 and/or mainly IgG at the epithelial basement membrane zone (but see other subepithelial vesiculobullous disorders). The lamina propria is diffusely infiltrated with mononuclear cells and eosinophils are prominent.

Management

Symptomatic patients usually respond to topical corticosteroids. An ophthalmological opinion is always indicated.

Erythema multiforme

Oral erythema multiforme (EM) is invariably symptomatic, causing intense soreness. It is far less common than LP and MMP and most affected patients are young adult males. EM is a recurrent disorder in which there are acute episodes of mouth ulcers and blood-stained crusting of the lips in over 40% of patients. Patients seen in oral medicine practice have oral lesions alone in 25–60%[5,6]: others have cutaneous lesions or involvement of other mucosae. Oral lesions occur mainly anteriorly in the mouth and especially affect the labial mucosa[5].

Clinical appearance

Vesicles or bullae (haemorrhagic) are rarely seen. Most patients present with an acute onset of swelling of the lips and/or tongue, with oral ulceration, and a serosanguinous exudate on the lips (Figure 1.5). There may be pyrexia, malaise, and/or cervical lymph node enlargement. Many, but not all, patients develop lesions on the skin or on the other mucosae.

Prognosis

The oral lesions are often recurrent but usually resolve after six or seven episodes within a mean period of 3 years (range 1–25). The periodicity of oral erythema multiforme can vary from weeks to years[5,6].

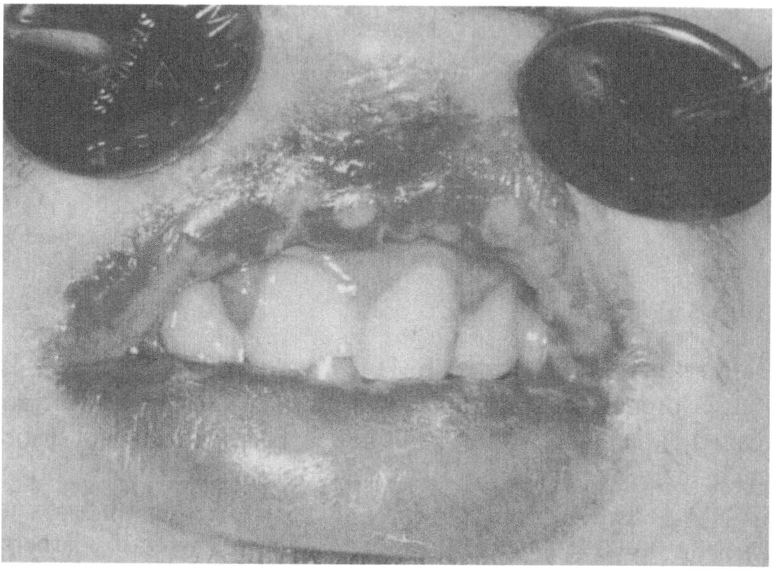

FIGURE 1.5 Erythema multiforme

Aetiology

The aetiology of oral EM, where definable, is similar to that of EM affecting other sites, viz. an immunological reaction to a range of agents such as herpes simplex virus, mycoplasma or drugs, but no precipitant can be identified in about 52% of cases[5].

Diagnosis

Diagnosis of oral EM is essentially by history and clinical appearance. Other vesiculobullous disorders (such as pemphigus and pemphigoid) and other oculomucocutaneous syndromes (Reiter's syndrome; Behçet's syndrome) may need to be excluded. Biopsy may be indicated where the appearance is not pathognomonic but is not always helpful, since sub- or intra-epithelial vesiculation may occur and pathology is very variable[7]. Immunostaining shows fibrin and C3 at the BMZ, and perivascular IgM, C3 and fibrin[8]. Inter- and/or intra-cellular oedema, acanthosis, irregular elongation of rete ridges, vasodilatation, oedema of the upper lamina propria, and perivascular mononuclear cell infiltration are the most obvious features but are rarely seen together[7]. Since differentiation from acute herpetic stomatitis can be difficult, virological studies may be indicated.

Management

Precipitating factors should be treated where possible and oral hygiene should be improved with 0.2% aqueous chlorhexidine mouthbaths. Supportive care is the mainstay, since specific treatment is not available. Corticosteroids *may* be indicated[5] with or without azathioprine[9]. Levamisole can be beneficial[10] and thalidomide has occasionally been used to some effect[11].

LESS COMMON SUBEPITHELIAL VESICULOBULLOUS DISORDERS

It has become apparent that a range of distinct disorders such as pemphigoid can result in subepithelial vesiculation; immunostaining of mucosal biopsies is invariably required to differentiate these, especially from dermatitis herpetiformis and linear IgA disease[3].

Bullous pemphigoid

Oral involvement is probably commoner in bullous pemphigoid than was formerly supposed: bullae and/or erosions are found in 8–49% of patients, and 80% of those with skin lesions alone have subclinical oral involvement[12]. Oral lesions appear to be commoner in those with negative indirect immunofluorescence[13,14] but have no influence on the prognosis or prevalence of associated malignancy[14].

Dermatitis herpetiformis and linear IgA disease

Dermatitis herpetiformis (DH) produces oral lesions in 4–70% of those with skin lesions[15,16], but IgA deposits are also detectable in clinically normal oral mucosa in up to 46% of cases[17–19]. Linear IgA disease may also produce oral lesions[19–21] and IgA deposits are also detectable in clinically normal oral mucosa[19]. Skin lesions usually, but not invariably, precede oral involvement[22].

Clinical appearance

Oral lesions of DH are erythematous, purpuric, or vesicular, affecting mainly the palate, buccal mucosa or gingiva[16]. Lesions of linear IgA disease are clinically similar in appearance and distribution[19–21].

Aetiology

Immune complexes involving IgA may be involved in the aetiology, though the presence of IgA deposits in uninvolved tissue casts doubt on its involvement. Gluten sensitivity may be involved[23].

Diagnosis

Diagnosis is by biopsy of oral lesions with immunostaining; serology is of little diagnostic value.

Management

Oral lesions tend to respond to systemic therapy using dapsone. It is unclear whether a gluten-free diet significantly influences the course of oral lesions.

SKIN DISEASES IN WHICH ORAL LESIONS MAY SIGNIFICANTLY CONTRIBUTE TO DIAGNOSIS

Oral lesions in LP, MMP, EM or other diseases can contribute to the diagnosis, but it is particularly in pemphigus and, to some extent, lupus erythematosus that oral lesions appear early, often as the presenting features, and can lead to an early diagnosis that facilitates management.

Pemphigus vulgaris

Oral lesions can be found in most types of pemphigus but are especially common in pemphigus vulgaris. Patients with pemphigus are usually late middle-aged or elderly, and females predominate. Oral lesions occur in most patients and are usually symptomatic ulcers; oral blisters are thin-walled and are thus rarely found intact[24,25]. Oral lesions in more than 60% of patients predate cutaneous lesions[25]. The skin lesions follow mouth lesions after 6–12 months.

Clinical appearance

Most patients present with persistent, irregular, ragged painful ulcers or erosions in any part of the mouth, but most commonly on the buccal and palatal mucosa (Figure 1.6). The Nikolsky sign is often positive. There is no scarring[26].

Prognosis

Oral lesions of pemphigus vulgaris are persistent, spread in the absence of treatment, and are often recalcitrant even when cutaneous lesions are controlled by treatment[26].

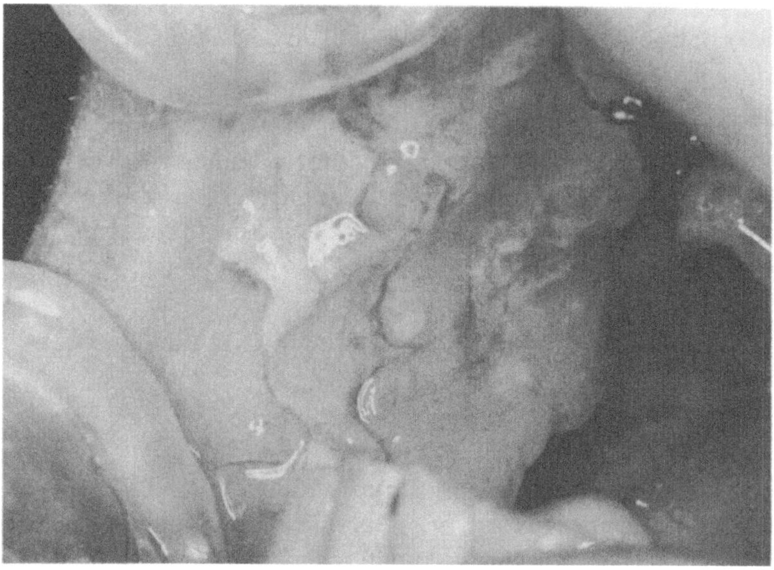

FIGURE 1.6 Pemphigus vulgaris

Aetiology

Pemphigus is an autoimmune disorder with a predilection for Arabs, Jews and others from the Mediterranean littoral.

Diagnosis

Although the history and clinical features may suggest pemphigus, a biopsy (with immunostaining) is essential and shows acantholysis and/or intercellular deposition of IgG and/or C3, though immunostaining may be negative in early disease[27]. Serum levels of antibody to epithelial intercellular cement show some relationship to disease activity but the correlation is not invariable[27] and some 25% of patients are seronegative[28]. Seronegativity is less likely if human rather than animal epithelium is used as substrate[29].

Oral smears for acantholytic cells are of little practical value. Apart from pemphigus, there are many other causes of oral ulceration, which are summarized in Table 1.3.

Management

High-dose corticosteroids with steroid-sparing agents such as azathioprine, levamisole, dapsone or gold are indicated[30–32].

Lupus erythematosus

Oral lesions occur both in discoid lupus erythematosus (DLE) and systemic lupus erythematosus (SLE)[33]. Oral lesions affect some 20–25% of those with DLE and 15–45% of those with SLE. Oral lesions of DLE occasionally precede cutaneous lesions of DLE and some 15% have SLE at presentation. A further 8% develop SLE later[33].

Clinical appearance

Oral lesions of DLE consist of a central area with white spots or papules radiating white striae at the margins and peripheral telangiectasia (Figure 1.7). Lesions of DLE attack mainly the buccal mucosa and vermilion of the lower lip – the latter are often crusted or scaly. About 15% of oral lesions of DLE progress to produce a leukoplakia – probably the counterpart of atrophic skin scars[33].

Oral lesions of SLE are usually discoid or erythematous lesions (occasionally ulcers), especially of the hard palate, buccal mucosa or vermilion of the lip.

Prognosis

Oral ulcers appear to occur most in those with DLE who will progress to SLE, and are more prevalent in those with active lupus. Oral lesions of SLE with IgG, C3 or IgA deposits on immunostaining are more likely than those with IgM alone to predict cutaneous and renal involvement[33]. Labial lesions of DLE, but not intra-oral lesions, have a small premalignant potential[33].

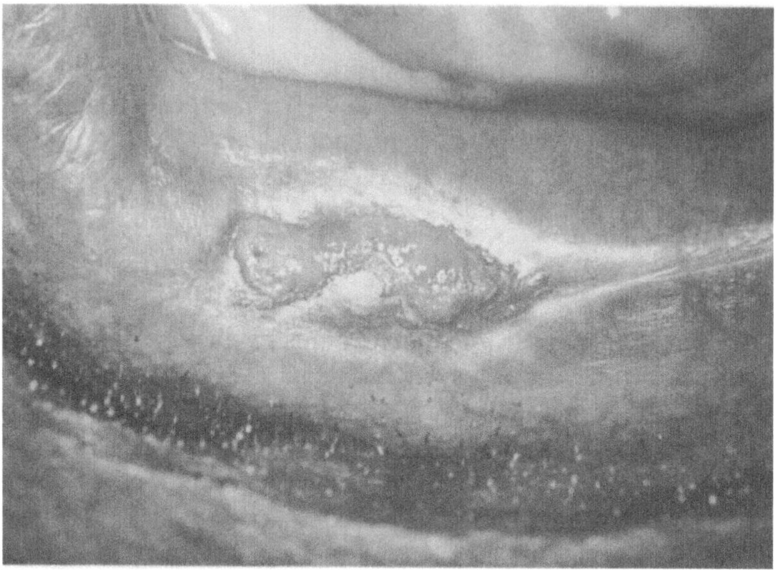

FIGURE 1.7 Discoid lupus erythematosus of the labial mucosa

Aetiology

The aetiology of LE is unclear but may involve the interplay of environmental, hormonal and viral factors with a host genetic predisposition[33].

Diagnosis

Clinical diagnosis of oral LE can be very difficult and differentiation from lichen planus in particular can be impossible. Biopsy is indicated and use of Lever's criteria of hyperkeratosis with keratotic plugs, atrophy of the stratum malpighii, hydropic degeneration in the basal cell layer, a patchy lymphoid infiltration in the lamina propria, and oedema with vasodilatation in the upper lamina propria, are useful in diagnosis. Granular deposits of IgM mainly (rather than IgG as in skin) are found at the basement membrane zone in most lesional and some 50% of apparently normal oral mucosa[33].

Management

Topical corticosteroids are effective in oral DLE but betamethasone *cream* rather than triamcinolone should be used. Isolated circumscribed lesions can effectively be excised or treated with cryosurgery. Recalcitrant lesions may respond to dapsone, antimalarials or systemic steroids. Oral lesions of SLE tend to respond to conventional systemic treatment of SLE[33].

Behçet's syndrome

Aphthous ulcers are characteristic features of Behçet's syndrome (BS). Patients are usually young or middle-aged adults; males predominate. Oral lesions may precede, accompany, or follow systemic lesions[34].

Clinical appearance

Mouth ulcers are found in virtually all patients with BS. The ulcers clinically and histologically so closely resemble recurrent aphthae that it is as yet impossible to define those few patients with aphthae who will progress to BS, unless systemic lesions are present (Figure 1.8).

Recurrent *aphthae* in BS may assume any of three clinical types, but the unifying features are recurrences and the onset in young adult life[34]. Minor aphthae are 2–4 mm in diameter, affect mainly the buccal or labial mucosa, and heal within 14 days, without scarring. Major aphthae are very much larger (> 1 cm), affect any site, and take 1 month or more to heal – often with scarring. Herpetiform ulcers start as multiple minute ulcers that enlarge to give ragged ulcers, anywhere on the mucosa, healing slowly, over a month or so.

Prognosis

The oral lesions can be difficult to control.

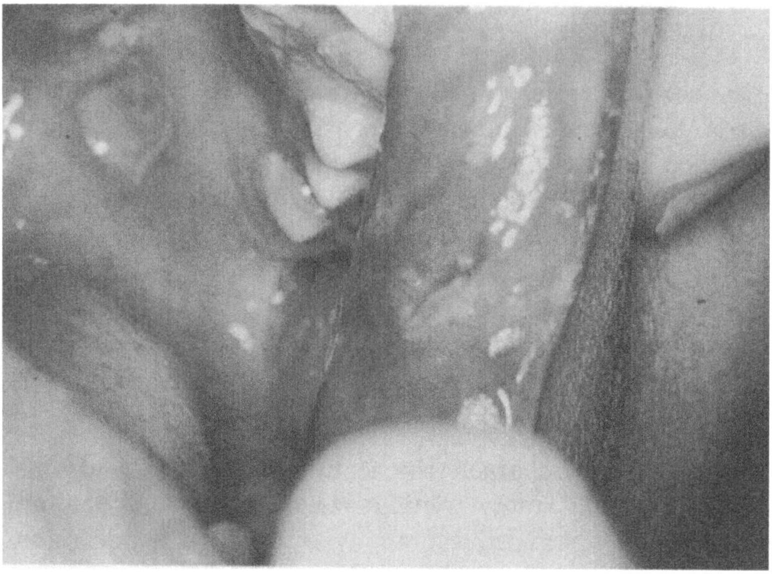

FIGURE 1.8 Typical aphthous-like oral ulceration of Behçet's syndrome

Aetiology

The aetiology of BS is unclear but may be viral[34].

Diagnosis

The diagnosis of BS is made on the basis of history and examination: there are no specific laboratory diagnostic investigations and pathergy (pustulation at the site of venepuncture) is uncommon in UK patients.

Management

BS may respond to topical corticosteroids or systemic treatment, such as with colchicine, dapsone or thalidomide[34].

Many of the less common disorders with both oral and cutaneous manifestations have an immunological basis (usually autoimmunity); these are summarized in Tables 1.6 and 1.7.

TABLE 1.6 Oral manifestations of immunologically-mediated skin diseases

Disease	*Oral manifestations*
Dermatitis herpetiformis (and linear IgA disease)	Erythematous, pseudovesicular or purpuric lesions or ulcers
Dermatomyositis	Telangiectasia, myopathy
Erythema multiforme	Ulcers, serosanguinous exudate on swollen lips
Lichen planus	White lesions, erosions, atrophy, desquamative gingivitis
Lupus erythematosus	Atrophic red lesions with white border; ulcers
Pemphigoid	
bullous	*Rarely*: Blisters, ulcers, desquamative gingivitis
mucous membrane	Blisters, ulcers, desquamative gingivitis
Pemphigus	Ulcers, blisters (rarely) Desquamative gingivitis (rarely)
Polyarteritis nodosa	Erythema, papules, nodules, ulcers
Psoriasis	*Rarely*: Minute yellowish ulcers, geographic tongue, diffuse erythema, pustules

DISEASES INVOLVING THE LIPS

Surprisingly few systemic or oral conditions affect the lips. Foremost among disorders affecting the vermilion are immunologically related diseases such as erythema multiforme, lupus erythematosus, scleroderma and contact cheilitis. Infections such as candidosis, recurrent herpes labialis and, rarely, syphilis, molluscum contagiosum and impetigo tend to involve the perioral skin somewhat more than the vermilion. Tumours such as squamous carcinoma, keratoacanthoma and basal cell carcinoma tend to occur at or close to the mucocutaneous junction: apart from squamous carcinoma, the latter

TABLE 1.7 Oral manifestations of immunodeficiency disorders that have frequent skin involvement

Disorder	*Manifestations*
HIV infection	Candidosis Herpesvirus infections Kaposi's sarcoma Hairy leukoplakia Xerostomia
Candidosis endocrinopathy syndrome	Chronic mucocutaneous candidosis
Graft versus host disease	Lichenoid lesions Sjögren's syndrome
Severe combined immunodeficiency	Candidosis (including CMC) Viral infections Oral ulceration Absent tonsils Recurrent sinusitis
Sex-linked agammaglobulinaemia	Cervical lymph node enlargement Oral ulceration Recurrent sinusitis Absent tonsils
Common variable immunodeficiency	Recurrent sinusitis Candidosis (including CMC)
Selective IgA deficiency	Tonsillar hyperplasia Oral ulceration Viral infections Parotitis
Di George syndrome	Abnormal facies Candidosis (including CMC) Viral infections Bifid uvula
Ataxia telangiectasia	Recurrent sinusitis Oral ulceration Facial and oral telangiectasia Cervical lymphomata Mask-like facial expression
Wiskott–Aldrich syndrome	Candidosis Viral infections Purpura
Hereditary angioedema	Swellings of face, mouth and pharynx
Chronic benign neutropenia	Oral ulceration Severe periodontitis

Disorder	Manifestations
Cyclic neutropenia	Oral ulceration Severe periodontitis Eczematous lesions of the face
Chronic granulomatous disease	Cervical lymph node enlargement and suppuration Candidosis (including CMC) Enamel hypoplasia Acute gingivitis Oral ulceration
Myeloperoxidase deficiency	Candidosis (including CMC)
Chediak–Higashi syndrome	Cervical lymph node enlargement Oral ulceration Severe periodontitis
Job's syndrome (Hyper IgE syndrome)	Abnormal facies

tumours are *rare* in the mouth. Generalized swelling of the lips occurs in some systemic conditions such as angioedema, sarcoidosis and Crohn's disease (Table 1.8). Much of these conditions are discussed in standard texts: this chapter deals predominantly with three of the

TABLE 1.8 Causes of swellings in the lips*

Localized swellings	*Diffuse swellings*
Mucocele	Oedema from trauma/infection
Tumours	
Salivary adenoma	Angioedema
Squamous carcinoma	Cheilitis glandularis
Keratoacanthoma	Lymphangioma/haemangioma
Other	
Cysts	Oral Crohn's disease
Infections	Sarcoidosis
Chancre	Cheilitis granulomatosa
Abscess	Melkersson–Rosenthal syndrome
Insect bite	Orofacial granulomatosis
Foreign body	

* There is wide individual and racial variation in lip morphology and size

more orally related disorders of relevance to dermatology, viz. angular cheilitis, herpes labialis and oral Crohn's disease.

Angular cheilitis

Angular cheilitis (angular cheilosis, angular stomatitis, or perleche) is a common condition, predominantly affecting elderly denture-wearing patients. Usually asymptomatic, affected patients may complain either of soreness of the angle of the mouth (commissures) or of the cosmetic defect of lines at the commissures.

Clinical appearance

Angular cheilitis presents as red linear lesions at each commissure (Figure 1.9). Almost invariably there is also denture-induced stomatitis beneath the upper denture, manifesting as a painless erythema in the denture-bearing area of the palate[35]. Rarely, the jaws are overclosed and give a nutcracker appearance to the patient in profile.

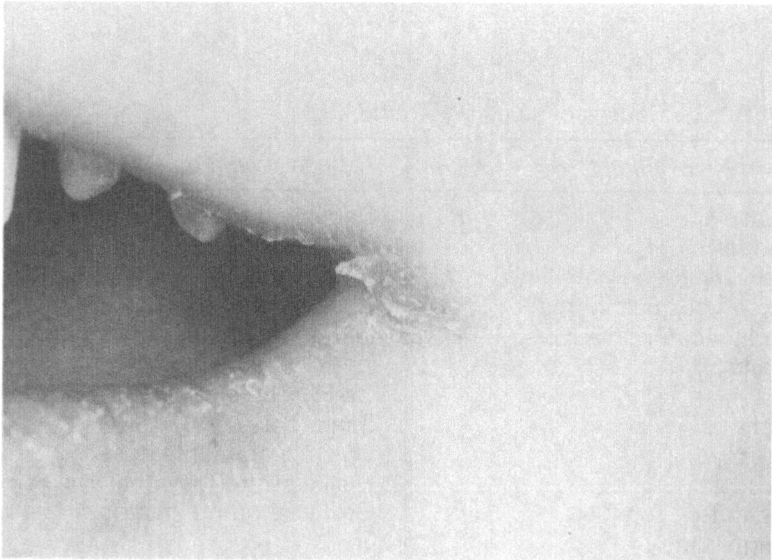

FIGURE 1.9 Angular cheilitis

Prognosis

In the absence of correct treatment, angular cheilitis often persists and deep painful fissures occasionally result.

Aetiology

In most instances, angular cheilitis is a complication of denture-induced stomatitis – a candida-induced lesion caused by poor denture hygiene and by wearing of dentures at night. It is caused by *Candida albicans*; other organisms such as staphylococci and streptococci may also be present in the commissural lesions.

Angular cheilitis that fails to resolve, or that occurs in patients who do not wear dentures, has more serious connotations. Deficiencies of iron, folate, or **B** vitamins (B_2, B_6, B_{12}) may rarely be implicated. A few patients prove to have oral Crohn's disease (see below). Angular cheilitis is also now recognized as one form of candidosis in HIV-infected patients (Table 1.9) and it can also occur in chronic muco-cutaneous candidosis.

TABLE 1.9 Causes of angular cheilitis

1.	Candidosis with denture-induced stomatitis
2.	Deficiency states
	Iron
	Folic acid
	Riboflavin
	Vitamin B_{12}
3.	Systemic disease
	Crohn's disease
	AIDS and related syndromes

Diagnosis

The diagnosis is invariably based on history and clinical examination alone.

Management

In that majority of cases associated with denture-wearing, angular cheilitis responds to leaving the dentures out of the mouth at night, storing them in hypochlorite, and treating the mucosal lesions with miconazole gel. In others, treatment of the underlying systemic disorder is also indicated.

Recurrent herpes labialis

Recurrent herpes labialis (RHL) affects up to 30% of those who have had a primary infection with herpes simplex virus (HSV)[34].

Clinical appearance

Vesiculation at or near the mucocutaneous junction follows a premonitory tingling or burning sensation. Vesicles become sterile pustules and scab to heal in 10 days to 3 weeks. Lesions may be haemorrhagic if there is a *bleeding tendency* as in leukaemia, and extensive if there is eczema or an immune defect.

Prognosis

Prognosis is good unless bacterial superinfection occurs. Recurrences are invariably frequent or severe.

Aetiology

HSV is latent in the trigeminal ganglion after primary infection. A transient immune defect is associated with RHL and the lesions can be frequent and severe if there is immunosuppression. Factors such as ultraviolet light, trauma, a concomitant febrile illness, immune defect, or menstruation can precipitate an episode of RHL[34].

Diagnosis

The diagnosis is clinical and usually straightforward. Occasionally zoster, impetigo or carcinoma can cause confusion and viral culture or electron microscopy of vesicular fluid is then helpful in diagnosis.

Management

Antivirals *if applied early* are valuable: acyclovir 5% cream is the preferred preparation. Immunocompromised patients may require systemic acyclovir[34].

Oral Crohn's disease

An uncommon cause of painless, chronic labial swelling is a chronic non-caseating granulomatous disorder that sometimes occurs in patients with Crohn's disease of the intestine, occasionally in sarcoidosis and, in other patients, appears to be confined to the mouth[36]. Conditions with a variety of titles such as Melkersson–Rosenthal syndrome, cheilitis granulomatosa (of Meischer) and, more recently, orofacial granulomatosis, appear to fall into this category (Table 1.8). Patients of either sex and any age, including children, are affected, the usual complaint being of the cosmetic problem.

Clinical appearance

Clinical features are variable in type but are usually chronic and can include:

1. Swelling(s) of lips and/or face (Figure 1.10)
2. Mucosal thickening and folding (cobblestoning), gingival hyperplasia and tags
3. Oral ulcers
4. Angular cheilitis
5. Lower motor neurone facial palsy

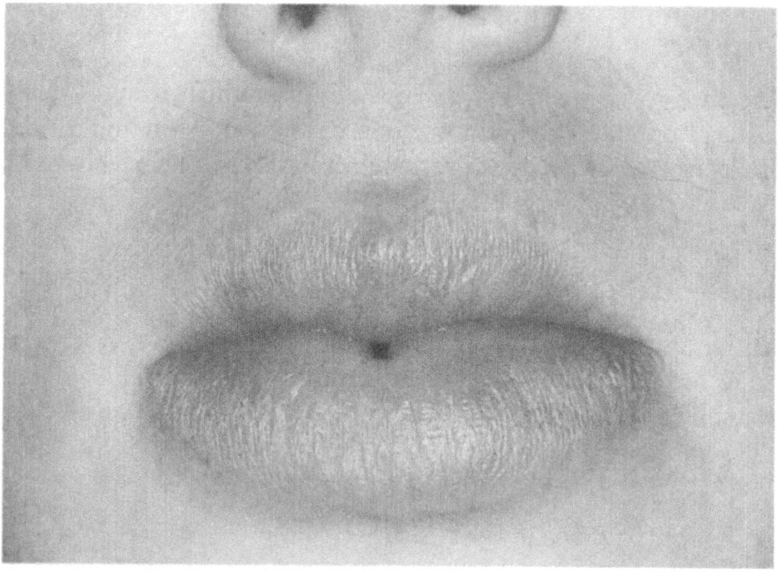

FIGURE 1.10 Oral Crohn's disease

The lips when swollen are erythematous and generally somewhat tender and often develop vertical fissures.

Prognosis

Orofacial lesions are persistent and recalcitrant to treatment.

Aetiology

The aetiology is unclear. A minority of patients prove to have intestinal Crohn's disease or sarcoidosis; even fewer have tuberculosis. Some are food-allergic and, in general, there is a higher prevalence of atopic disease in this group of patients than in the normal population.

Diagnosis

The history and examination are of major importance and the most useful investigation is a deep lesional biopsy. Crohn's disease and sarcoidosis should be excluded by conventional examination and investigations.

Management

It can be worth giving a trial of an antigen-free or low-antigen diet, but the labial swelling may only respond to intralesional corticosteroids.

REFERENCES

1. Scully, C. and Elkom, M. (1985). Lichen planus: Review and update on pathogenesis. *J. Oral Pathol.*, **14,** 431–8.
2. Silverman, S. Jr., Gorsky, M., Lozada-Nur, F. and Liv, A. (1986). Oral mucous membrane pemphigoid. A study of sixty-five patients. *Oral Surg.*, **61,** 233–7.
3. Williams, D. M., Leonard, J. N., Wright, P., Gilkes, J. J. H., Haffendum, G. P., McMinn, R. M. H. and Fry, L. (1984). Benign mucous membrane (cicatricial) pemphigoid revisited: a clinical and immunological reappraisal. *Br. Dent. J.*, **157,** 313–16.
4. Stephenson, P., Lamey, P. J., Scully, C. and Prime, S. S. (1987). Angina bullosa haemorrhagica – clinical and laboratory features in 30 patients. *Oral Surg.*, **63,** 560–5.
5. Lozada, F. and Silverman, S. (1978). Erythema multiforme. *Oral Surg.*, **46,** 628–36.
6. Leigh, I. M., Mowbray, J. F., Levene, G. M. and Sutherland, S. (1985). Recurrent and continuous erythema multiforme – a clinical and immunological study. *Clin. Exp. Dermatol.*, **10,** 58–67.
7. Buchner, A., Lozada, F. and Silverman, S. (1980). Histopathologic spectrum of oral erythema multiforme. *Oral Surg.*, **49,** 221–8.
8. Howland, W. W., Golitz, L. E., Weston, W. L. and Huff, J. C. (1984). Erythema multiforme: clinical, histopathologic, and immunologic study. *J. Am. Acad. Dermatol.*, **10,** 438–46.
9. Lozada, F. (1981). Prednisone and azathioprine in the treatment of patients with vesiculoerosive oral diseases. *Oral Surg.*, **53,** 257–60.
10. Lozada, F. (1982). Levamisole in the treatment of erythema multiforme. A double-blind trial in fourteen patients. *Oral Surg.*, **53,** 28–31.
11. Bahmer, F. A., Zaun, H. and Luszpinski, P. (1983). Thalidomide treatment of recurrent erythema multiforme. *Acta Dermatovener (Stockholm)*, **62,** 449–50.
12. Laskaris, G. and Nicolis, G. (1980). Immunopathology of oral mucosa in bullous pemphigoid. *Oral Surg.*, **50,** 340–5.
13. Person, J. R. and Rogers, R. S. (1977). Bullous and cicatricial pemphigoid clinical, histopathologic and immunopathologic correlations. *Mayo Clin. Proc.*, **52,** 54–7.
14. Hodge, L., Marsden, R. A., Black, M. M., Bhogal, B. and Corbett, M. F. (1981).

Bullous pemphigoid; the frequency of mucosal involvement and for concurrent malignancy related to indirect immunofluorescence findings. *Br. J. Dermatol.*, **105,** 65–9.
15. Katz, S. I. (1978). Dermatitis herpetiformis: clinical, histologic, therapeutic and laboratory clues. *Int. J. Dermatol.*, **17,** 529–35.
16. Fraser, N. G., Kerr, N. W. and Donald, D. (1973). Oral lesions in dermatitis herpetiformis. *Br. J. Dermatol.*, **89,** 439–50.
17. Harrison, P. V., Scott, D. G. and Cobden, I. (1980). Buccal mucosa immunofluorescence in coeliac disease and dermatitis herpetiformis. *Br. J. Dermatol.*, **102,** 687–8.
18. Nisengard, R. J., Chorzelski, T., Maciejowska, E. and Kryst, L. (1982). Dermatitis herpetiformis; IgA deposits in gingiva, buccal mucosa, and skin. *Oral Surg.*, **54,** 22–5.
19. Hietanen, J. and Reunala, T. (1984). IgA deposits in the oral mucosa of patients with dermatitis herpetiformis and linear IgA disease. *Scand. J. Dent. Res.*, **92,** 230–4.
20. Wiesenfeld, D., Martin, A., Scully, C. and Thomson, J. (1982). Oral manifestations in linear IgA disease. *Br. Dent. J.*, **153,** 398–9.
21. Flotte, T. J., Olbricht, S. M., Collins, A. B. and Harrist, T. J. (1985). Immunopathologic studies of adult linear IgA bullous dermatosis. *Arch. Pathol. Lab. Med.*, **109,** 457–9.
22. Economopoulou, P. and Laskaris, G. (1986). Dermatitis herpetiformis: oral lesions as an early manifestation. *Oral Surg.*, **62,** 77–80.
23. Katz, S. I. and Strober, W. (1978). The pathogenesis of dermatitis herpetiformis. *J. Invest. Dermatol.*, **70,** 63–75.
24. Pisanti, S., Sharon, F. and Kaufman, E. (1974). Pemphigus vulgaris: incidence in Jews of different ethnic groups, according to age, sex, and initial lesion. *Oral Surg.*, **38,** 382–7.
25. Rosenburg, F. R., Sanders, S. and Nelson, C. T. (1976). Pemphigus: a 20 year review of 107 patients treated with corticosteroids. *Arch. Dermatol.*, **112,** 962–70.
26. Meurer, M., Millns, J. L., Rogers, R. S. and Jordan, R. E. (1977). Oral pemphigus vulgaris. *Arch. Dermatol.*, **113,** 1520–4.
27. Acosta, E., Gilkes, J. J. H. and Ivanyi, L. (1985). Relationship between the serum antibody titres and the clinical activity of pemphigus vulgaris. *Oral Surg.*, **60,** 611–14.
28. Judd, K. P. and Lever, W. F. (1979). Correlation of antibodies in skin and serum with disease severity in pemphigus. *Arch. Dermatol.*, **115,** 428–32.
29. Laskaris, G. (1981). Oral pemphigus vulgaris, an immunofluorescent study of fifty-eight cases. *Oral Surg.*, **51,** 626–31.
30. Lozada, F., Silverman, S. and Cram, D. (1982). Pemphigus vulgaris, a study of six cases treated with levamisole and prednisone. *Oral Surg.*, **54,** 161–5.
31. Haim, S. and Friedman-Bisbaum, R. (1978). Dapsone in the treatment of pemphigus vulgaris. *Dermatologica*, **186,** 120–3.
32. Lever, W. F. and Schaumburg-Lever, G. (1977). Immunosuppressants and prednisone in pemphigus vulgaris. Therapeutic results obtained in 63 patients between 1961 and 1975. *Arch. Dermatol.*, **113,** 1236–41.
33. Schiodt, M. (1984). Oral manifestations of lupus erythematosus. *Int. J. Oral Surg.*, **13,** 1–52.

34. Scully, C. and Porter, S. R. (1988). Oral manifestations of disorders of immunity. In Jones, J. H. and Mason, D. K. (eds.) *Oral manifestations of systemic disease*, 2nd Ed. (Eastbourne: W. B. Saunders)
35. Scully, C. (1986). Chronic atrophic candidosis (Leading Article). *Lancet*, **2,** 437–8.
36. Wiesenfeld, D., Ferguson, M. M., Mitchell, D. N., MacDonald, D. G., Scully, C., Cochran, K. and Russell, R. I. (1985). Orofacial granulomatosis: clinical and pathological analysis. *Q. J. Med.*, **213,** 101–13.

2

THE EYE AND THE SKIN

P. WRIGHT

BLEPHARITIS[1–4]

Lid margin inflammation (Table 2.1) is a common ophthalmic problem and in the USA it is said to account for 500 000 patient visits per year.

The classical pre-antibiotic, pre-steroid concept of blepharitis ascribed one-third of cases to seborrhoea, one-third to staphylococcal infection, and the remaining one-third were thought to have a mixed seborrhoeic-infective aetiology. Improved personal hygiene, potent topical antibiotics and steroids have changed the pattern of disease seen, and recent work has shown the strong dermatological associations of the main forms of lid margin inflammation.

Many factors influence the occurrence of each variant in a community, but climate is probably the most important, staphylococcal and seborrhoeic blepharitis occurring most often in

TABLE 2.1 Classification of blepharitis (after McCulley *et al.*)[1]

1. Staphylococcal
2. Seborrhoeic
   (a) pure seborrhoea
   (b) with staphylococcal superinfection
   (c) with meibomian seborrhoea
   (d) with secondary meibomian gland inflammation
3. Primary meibomian gland inflammation and meibomian kerato-conjuctivitis
4. Other (atopic, psoriatic, fungal, demodectic and parasitic)

warmer climates whilst meibomian kerato-conjuctivitis is a disease of cooler climes.

Staphylococcal blepharitis causes intermittent inflammation of the lid margin with crusting of the lashes and folliculitis of lash follicles leading to destruction of follicles and loss of eyelashes (madarosis) (Figure 2.1). The patients are mostly young, and symptoms and signs wax and wane. The skin is normal in 95% of cases with only a few having evidence of staphylococcal skin lesions elsewhere or microbiological evidence of staphylococcal carriage. Both coagulase-negative staphylococci and *Staphylococcus aureus* can be cultured from affected lids. *Staph. aureus* predominates in cases with folliculitis and madarosis.

Seborrhoeic blepharitis is a more chronic and persistent problem without signs of inflammation but with oily, greasy crusting of the lid margin and little disturbance of lash growth (Figure 2.2). Exacerbations occur with signs of inflammation as a result of secondary bacterial infection, usually with coagulase-negative staphylococci. This group of patients all show some evidence of seborrhoeic dermatitis, usually mild and limited to scalp and retro-auricular areas.

Meibomian gland disease. The meibomian glands are a series of

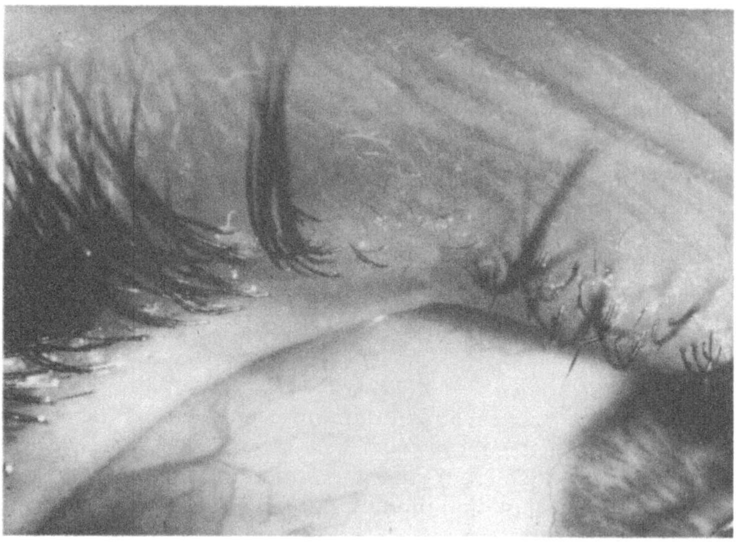

FIGURE 2.1 Staphylococcal blepharitis with loss of lashes

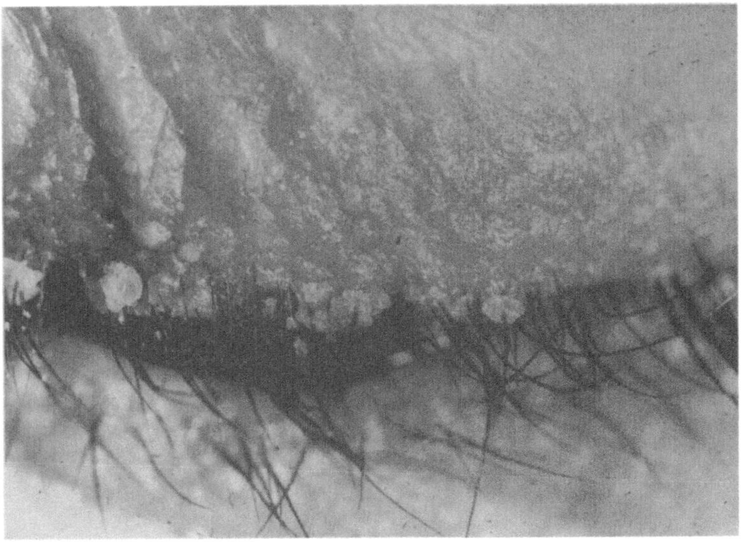

FIGURE 2.2 Seborrhoeic blepharitis with greasy crusting

glands lying within the substance of the lid and opening on to the lid margins. They produce a complex mixture of lipids, meibum, comparable to sebum but differing in composition. The lipid secreted by the glands floats as a monolayer on the precorneal tear fluid, stabilizing the fluid film and preventing evaporation. Disordered meibum production occurs either as a result of breakdown of the secretion by bacterial lipases or by an irritant effect on the epithelial lining of the terminal portion of the gland ductule adjacent to the lid margin. The organisms commonly recovered from the lids and glands are coagulase-negative staphylococci and proprionibacteria. Staphylococci produce three lipolytic enzymes: triglyceride lipase, fatty wax esterase and cholesteryl esterase. Proprionibacteria produce the first two enzymes but not cholesteryl esterase. The epithelial cells become keratinized and are shed into the duct lumen so that expression of the glands yields opaque toothpaste-like material rather than the clear yellowish oily material normally produced (Figure 2.3). Complete obstruction of the lumen may occur and causes the development of a sterile lipogranuloma known as a chalazion or meibomian cyst (Figure 2.4). Florid meibomitis is associated with severe keratoconjunctivitis in which sterile peripheral corneal infiltrates develop

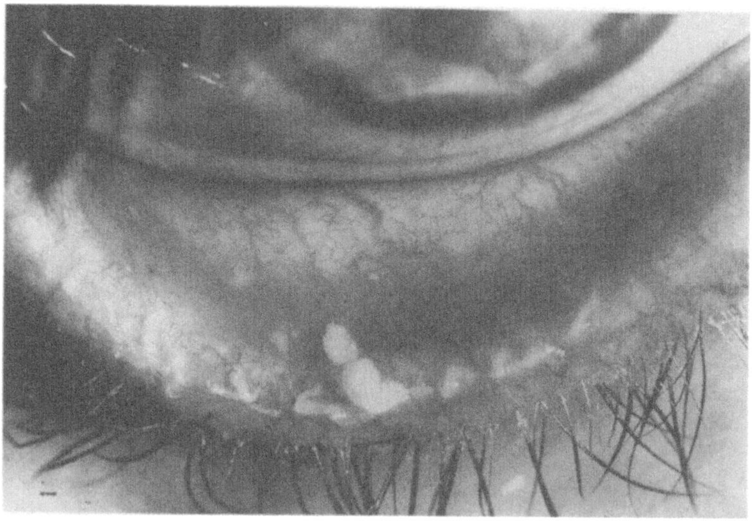

FIGURE 2.3 Obstructed meibomian glands and opaque secretion

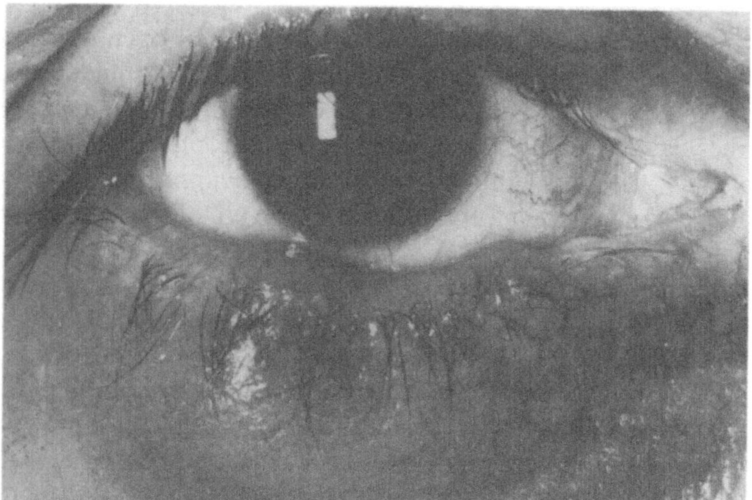

FIGURE 2.4 Meibomian cysts associated with acne rosacea

with corneal thinning and vascularization. The more advanced cases of meibomian kerato-conjunctivitis show identical changes to those seen in acne rosacea and certainly acne rosacea is the major skin finding associated with meibomitis. As many as 95% of patients with meibomitis are said to show some evidence of acne rosacea, but widely differing figures are quoted for different populations and geographical areas.

Meibomian seborrhoea is a less clear-cut entity in which excessive secretion is produced, probably of altered composition, which produces chronic burning and irritation of the eyes without many objective signs. The eyes tend to be red, with hyperaemic conjunctiva but no other signs of inflammation. Foam is seen along the edge of the lids as a result of altered surface activity of the tear lipid mixture. A variable but smaller number of these patients show associated skin changes, either seborrhoea or acne rosacea.

Treatment of blepharitis

Blepharitis is probably best regarded as a chronic disorder without cure but permitting of some control and amelioration. Treatment can be vigorous in the acute phase, with lid margin toilet and topical antibiotics. Chloramphenicol ointment 1% remains the most frequently prescribed and gives fewer problems of contact sensitivity than the aminoglycosides such as neomycin or gentamicin. Chronic cases need lid swabs to determine the strains present and sensitivity of the organisms, since resistant strains quickly develop. Treatment of associated seborrhoea, especially of the scalp, is usually advised but probably gives little benefit. Topical steroid/antibiotic ointment combinations are frequently prescribed for seborrhoeic blepharitis but give only transient relief of symptoms and carry an unacceptably high risk of steroid adverse effects in those patients who have chronic symptoms. Lens opacities, secondary glaucoma and potentiation of viral and other infections are the major sight-threatening complications of long-term use of steroid ointments and drops. Seborrhoeic blepharitis, however troublesome, is never sight-threatening.

Meibomitis does not respond to topical antibiotics but responds well to oral tetracycline or erythromycin in a low-dose régime, 250 mg b.d., whether classical skin changes of acne rosacea are present or not. Trimethoprim–sulphonamide combinations or cephalosporins may be required for chronic cases or when lid swabs show organisms (usually coagulase-negative staphylococci) resistant to tetracycline and erythromycin. Chalazia and meibomian cysts require surgical incision and curettage, a minor procedure done under local anaesthesia. The corneal complications of meibomian kerato-conjunctivitis are indistinguishable from those of acne rosacea and are treated similarly.

ACNE ROSACEA[5]

Ocular complications of acne rosacea have been recognized for over a hundred years, but not all patients with facial rosacea develop ocular symptoms or signs and the ocular features may develop with minimal or absent skin changes.

The ocular complications can involve all the structures of the outer eye with blepharitis, conjunctivitis, scleritis and sclerokeratitis. Many of these changes are indistinguishable from blepharitis and the changes associated with chronic staphylococcal lid margin infection (staphylococcal hypersensitivity syndrome).

Rosacea blepharitis typically involves the meibomian glands and is of the type in which plugging of the meibomian orifices occurs with white cheesey material on expression of the affected glands and repeated meibomian cyst or chalazion formation. The lid margins become thickened and there may be dilated telangiectatic vessels present on the skin, but more often on the transitional zone of the lid edge between skin and conjunctiva (Figure 2.5). Scarring and plugging of the meibomian orifices also make the lid edge irregular, and distortion of the tarsal plate caused by tarsal conjunctival inflammation causes the lid to turn slightly inwards, producing first degree entropion with the abnormal meibomian orifices pointing backwards in upper and lower lids to rub against the ocular surface. This structural alteration of the lid/globe contact brings the abnormal meibomian material and any bacteria present into intimate contact with the ocular surface, overcoming some of the normal barriers of the ocular

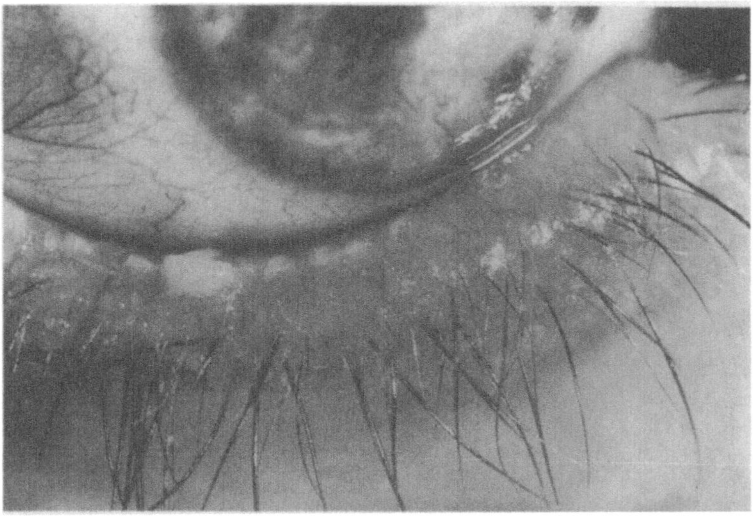

FIGURE 2.5 Dilated vessels and metaplasia of lid margin in acne rosacea

mucus and tear layers. Conjunctival hyperaemia without evidence of infection and, again, dilated telangiectatic vessels may be seen in the bulbar conjunctiva, especially inferiorly in the pericorneal region. Scleral and episcleral inflammation with nodules may occur and may progress to scleral thinning but never to necrosis or perforation (Figure 2.6). Sclerokeratitis is commoner and is a major sight-threatening complication of acne rosacea. The typical lesions are marginal corneal infiltrates, pale yellow in colour, occurring in the lower nasal or lower temporal quadrants and associated with only localized epithelial breakdown or ulceration. The epithelium may remain intact over the infiltrates. The sclera adjacent to the corneal inflammation is often involved, hence the descriptive term sclerokeratitis. Microbiological examination of the corneal lesions shows no bacteria but numerous inflammatory cells, and the lesions are thought to be due to a sterile, cell-mediated immune response. Untreated, the inflammation extends to involve progressively more and more central areas of the cornea. Spontaneous improvement can occur but is followed by further waves of inflammation at the head of the original lesion, so that scarring progresses steadily toward the central cornea. As the lesions extend, the cornea becomes thinned and vascularized. Peripheral lesions cause

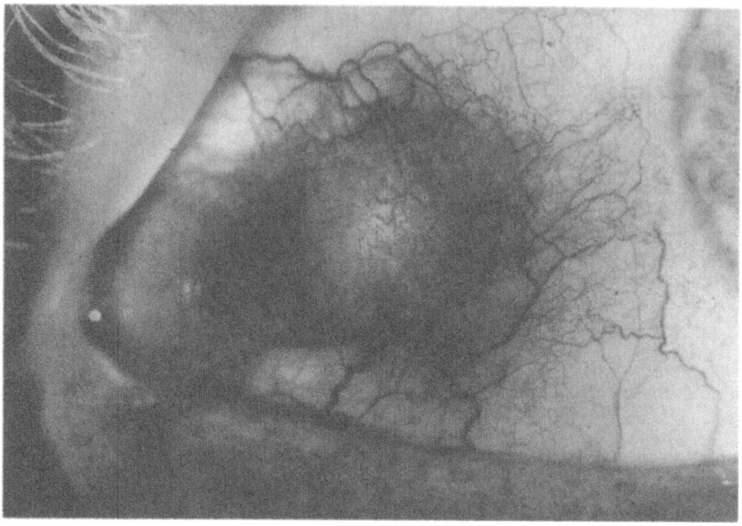

FIGURE 2.6 Episcleral nodule in acne rosacea

pain and photophobia and vision may be impaired by astigmatism resulting from corneal irregularity. Involvement of the central cornea results in profound visual loss (Figure 2.7).

Treatment of the blepharitis is as previously described for meibomitis, with oral antibiotics. The sclerokeratitis requires treatment with both oral tetracycline or erythromycin and topical steroids. Topical antibiotics have no place since the corneal lesions are sterile. Long-term steroids are contra-indicated because of the risks of steroid glaucoma, cataract and potentiation of viral and fungal infections. Most patients relapse if treatment is withdrawn too quickly and many need treatment with low-dose oral antibiotics over several years. The tetracycline alone by mouth, 250 mg once or twice a day, is often sufficient to control recurrences of keratitis. It is believed to act by blocking inflammatory cell recruitment and by its anticomplementary activity in addition to the antibacterial effects. Late complications of the keratitis include lipid deposition in the scarred areas, and perforation of the thinned cornea may occur. Lipid deposition clears if the peripheral corneal vessels are occluded by laser, but the vessels may be difficult to visualize and exacerbations of sclerokeratitis and more corneal thinning may follow the laser treatment. Central corneal

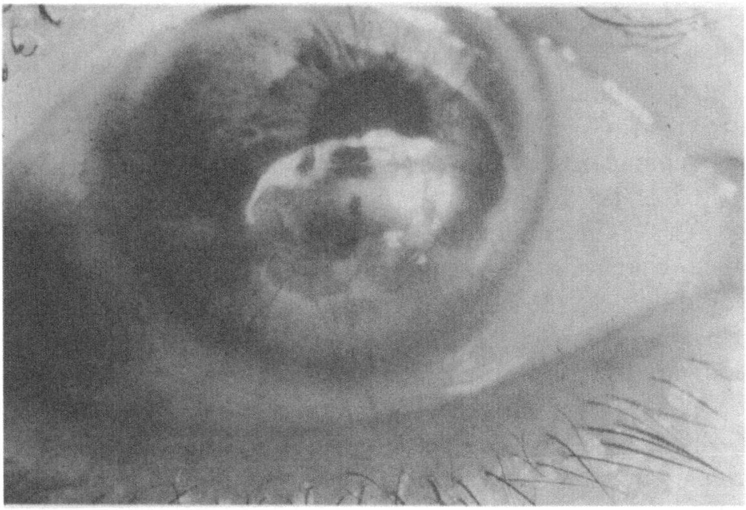

FIGURE 2.7 Rosacea keratitis

scarring may require treatment by corneal transplantation, but the surgery can be technically difficult because of irregularity and thinning of the recipient cornea and recurrences of rosacea keratitis occur in the graft if the condition is not generally controlled.

ALLERGIC EYE DISEASE

Atopic individuals can manifest a number of patterns of inflammation of the outer eye, including blepharitis, periorbital eczema, conjunctivitis and keratitis of various types.

Allergic blepharitis other than due to contact sensitivity to applied topical medication is rare. Patients with facial eczema tend to have periorbital changes and the lids become thickened and excoriated. The thickening of the anterior lamella of the lid can cause ectropion leading to epiphora and further excoriation of the skin. The abnormal lid margins become infected with staphylococci, often *Staph. aureus*, and some of the associated conjunctival changes are believed to be due to a secondary hypersensitivity to the bacterial exotoxins or other disordered products of lid margin glands as described in the section on blepharitis.

Allergic conjunctivitis may be acute or chronic. Acute allergic conjunctivitis is typically seen as part of the hay fever group of disorders and is characterized by intense itching and watering of the eyes with swelling of the conjunctiva, which may bulge out between the lids (chemosis). The swelling is usually transient and not associated with corneal changes or visual impairment, although the symptoms may be disabling.

Chronic allergic conjunctivitis is almost always a kerato-conjunctivitis, i.e. corneal changes develop and are secondary to the chronic inflammation of the conjunctiva lining the lids. Two clinically distinct patterns emerge, the condition in childhood known as vernal conjunctivitis or spring catarrh, and the adult disease which is adult atopic kerato-conjunctivitis.

Vernal conjunctivitis was so called because it shows periodic activity, mainly in the spring but also at other times of the year, especially autumn. It occurs in all parts of the world and has differing clinical features in different geographic areas, with varying degrees of involvement of the lid or globe conjunctiva and the cornea. Other evidence of atopy (eczema, asthma, or elevated serum IgE) is found in one-third of cases. A further one-third give a close family history of atopic disease, whilst the remaining one-third are non-atopes. The condition begins in childhood, usually before the age of seven, and mostly improves and remits spontaneously before or at puberty. The seasonal exacerbations may be associated with spring flower pollen and with tree pollen in the autumn, but patch testing and desensitization are of little value in management of the conjunctival disorder even when helpful in treating other allergic manifestations such as asthma that may be associated. The affected children develop lid swelling, itching and watery mucoid discharge containing numerous eosinophils. The lids may become heavy and droop (ptosis). The mucoid discharge greatly increases when the condition is active and the eyes become red, with some degree of chemosis. The conjunctival changes mainly affect the upper tarsal conjunctiva in the palpebral form of the disease and the lower fornix may appear surprisingly normal. The upper tarsal conjunctiva can be examined after everting the lid by applying external pressure with a rod, matchstick or cotton bud to the surface of the upper part of the lid with one hand and then grasping the lashes with the fingers of the other hand to pull the lid away from the globe and upwards. The lid folds back on itself to reveal the tarsal conjunctiva. The patient is instructed to look steadily downward to relax the orbicularis oculi whilst carrying out the manœuvre, and at the end of the examination the lid will return to its usual position as the patient simply looks upward. Lid closure or failure to gaze steadily downward make it difficult or impossible to evert the lid.

The tarsal conjunctiva develops a diffuse pattern of papillary hypertrophy in all forms of chronic allergic eye disease, but in vernal conjunctivitis the giant compound hypertrophic papillae can become very large and impressive and are often described as cobble stones (Figure 2.8). When actively inflamed, the papillae are tightly packed together and the outlines are blurred by the tenacious mucoid discharge produced by the conjunctiva. When the inflammation is controlled, the papillae appear drier and harder, free from the covering mucoid material. Despite their formidable appearance, such papillae are asymptomatic and cause no mechanical damage to the cornea or bulbar conjunctiva. In addition to the inflammation of the tarsal

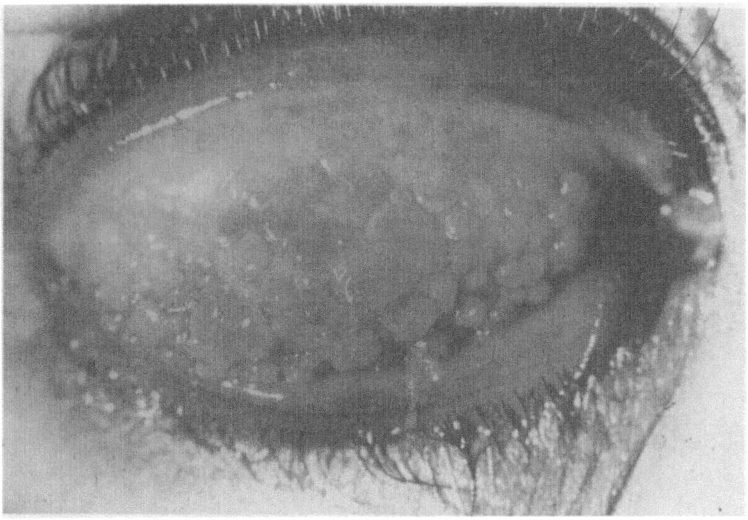

FIGURE 2.8 Vernal conjunctivitis (cobble stones)

conjunctiva, bulbar conjunctival changes can also occur. These may develop in association with tarsal changes or in isolation and the bulbar variant of the condition is seen more often in some geographical areas such as the West Indies and Middle East.

The bulbar form of vernal conjunctivitis presents with itchy, red eyes and watery discharge but not the heavy stringy mucoid discharge seen in palpebral vernal conjunctivitis. White swellings (limbal follicles) develop around the corneo-scleral junction and may be associated with clear spaces and cystic areas containing yellow granular material (Trantas' spots). The yellow material is believed to be eosinophil debris. The limbal changes most often develop superiorly but can occur at any point around the cornea or involve the whole limbal area (Figure 2.9). Corneal complications only develop if the conjunctival inflammation persists uncontrolled for some time.

Palpebral and limbal vernal conjunctivitis is never sight-impairing, but the corneal complications can cause significant visual loss. The earliest sign of keratitis is a greyness of the corneal epithelium, mainly involving the upper one third to one half of the cornea and progressing to epithelial breakdown. The eroded area of cornea is usually horizontally oval and on the base of the erosion is deposited mucus and

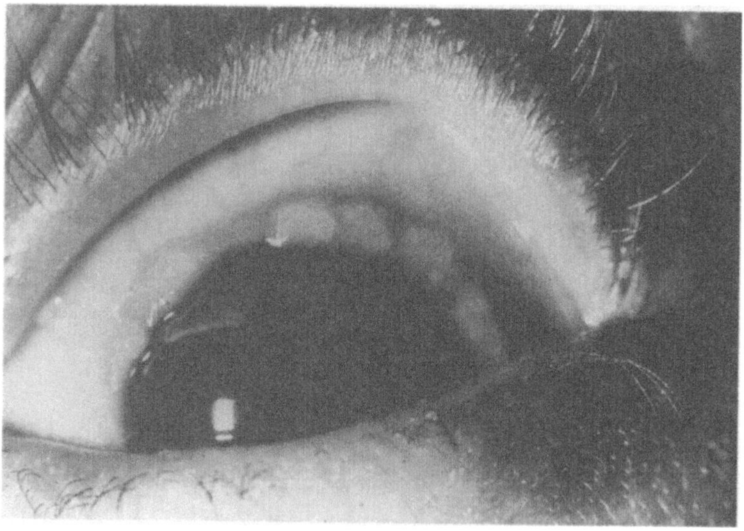

FIGURE 2.9 Bulbar vernal showing limbal follicles

fibrin to form a vernal plaque. These can persist almost indefinitely if the conjunctival inflammation is not controlled and successive waves of plaque formation can occur with periodic exacerbations of conjunctival inflammation.

Treatment of vernal conjunctivitis is with topical disodium cromoglycate (DSCG) and steroids. The conjunctiva in vernal conjunctivitis is full of mast cells and eosinophils in the active stage of the disease, but, despite the pharmacological specificity of cromones for this type of cellular infiltration, the response to DSCG is disappointing. Fewer than 20% of all cases of vernal conjunctivitis can be controlled with DSCG alone and these are only the mildest cases. Bulbar vernal conjunctivitis responds better than palpebral.

It follows that for all but the mildest cases topical steroid drops are required and, because of the difficulty in monitoring intra-ocular pressure in children, the weakest steroid that will just control the inflammation should be employed. Some commercial steroids such as clobetasone and fluorometholone have reduced potential to increase intra-ocular pressure but often prove too weak for very active inflammation.

At Moorfields we employ a semi-log dilution series of prednisolone drops with 1% as the strongest, then 0.3%, 0.1%, 0.03%, 0.01% and so on down. This allows a tailoring of the potency of the steroid treatment to the amount of inflammation present and greatly helps to reduce side-effects. For severe inflammation, especially when corneal complications develop, the highest concentration may be needed frequently, but steadily weaker drops can be substituted as the condition comes under control. Once controlled with dilute steroid, DSCG alone may prove sufficient to keep the conjunctiva quiet, especially during the cooler months. Topical antihistamine drops and vasoconstrictors are of no benefit and oral mast cell and basophil-stabilizing agents do not help. Vernal plaque requires intensive control of the conjunctival changes followed by careful surgical excision of the plaque. The epithelium can then grow back over the bare corneal surface and, provided that the surface is not too irregular, useful vision is recovered. Corneal transplants do badly in this group of patients and are avoided if possible. Surgical ablation of the giant papillae and treatments such as diathermy or cryotherapy of the conjunctiva are of no value. The papillae rapidly reform and the corneal changes, caused by the outpouring of mediators from inflamed conjunctiva, continue unabated.

Adult atopic kerato-conjunctivitis is a more chronic disease with periodic exacerbations that may coincide with worsening of the atopic manifestations generally or may occur in isolation. Lid thickening with ectropion occurs as previously described with secondary bacterial infection of the excoriated skin. The conjunctiva develops a papillary reaction that involves both upper and lower tarsal conjunctiva. The papillae are smaller and more regular than in vernal conjunctivitis and giant cobble stones are rarely seen (Figure 2.10). An associated epithelial keratitis develops in almost all cases and is associated with a moderate and variable amount of disturbance of vision depending upon the extent of involvement of the central area of the cornea. Bacterial corneal ulceration from spillover of lid infection and superficial vascularization occur in poorly controlled cases. With long-standing conjunctival inflammation the surface of the palpebral conjunctiva becomes metaplastic, losing its normal highly organized pattern with goblet cells to become a keratinized non-wettable squamous epithelium. Such changes inflict further damage on an already compromised corneal epithelium. Fine fibrosis forming a reticular

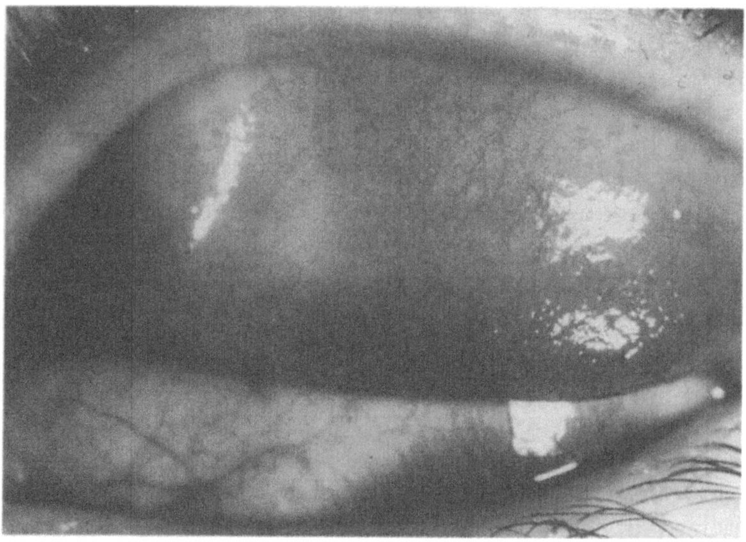

FIGURE 2.10 Adult atopic conjunctivitis

pattern also develops beneath the conjunctiva around the base of the papillae and is a unique diagnostic feature of atopic conjunctivitis. The squamous metaplasia also affects the lacrimal drainage system, causing narrowing or obstruction that worsens the epiphora and excoriation of the lids. The lacrimal obstruction in this group of patients is difficult to treat surgically.

Treatment of the condition generally is equally difficult. There is almost never any response to DSCG and topical steroids are the mainstay of treatment. High-potency steroids frequently instilled are needed and still do not control all features, the keratitis being particularly resistant to treatment. Squamous metaplasia once developed does not improve with control of the inflammation and topical retinoic acid, which has proved of value in dealing with other forms of conjunctival metaplasia, has not helped these atopic patients. Oral antibiotics such as tetracycline and erythromycin do help, possibly by controlling bacterial lid infection but more probably by exerting a direct anti-inflammatory effect on the conjunctiva as previously described for rosacea. The combination of impaired cellular immunity, need for high-potency steroids and risk of superadded bacterial and fungal infection make this group of patients one of the most difficult to treat of all external eye disease.

Systemic steroids are rarely indicated for the ocular features alone, but immunosuppression with steroids and cytotoxic agents such as azathioprine have improved ocular symptoms and signs when given for control of eczema, allowing reduced ocular topical therapy.

THE BULLOUS DERMATOSES[6–9]

Both pemphigus and the subepidermal dermatoses are associated with ocular changes. Whilst all can cause conjunctival inflammation, pemphigus causes no conjunctival scarring, but the others do in varying degrees.

Pemphigus vulgaris is associated with episodes of conjunctival inflammation that tend to occur with flares of the skin blistering. The conjunctiva, particularly that of the lids, becomes very red and swollen. The eyes are usually watery but secondary bacterial infection with discharge may occur. The palpebral conjunctiva appears thick and velvety with intense congestion. Fluorescein does not stain the surface of the conjunctiva and even with prolonged inflammation there is no breakdown or ulceration of the surface. The inflammation is very responsive to topical steroid therapy such as prednisolone drops and also responds to increased systemic treatment. Repeated attacks can occur without any long-term changes in the conjunctiva, but repeated eversion of the lids to examine the conjunctiva easily produces a positive Nikolsky sign in the skin of the lid.

Pemphigus foliaceus is said to have a higher incidence of ocular complications, especially corneal scarring, but the disease is rare and the limited descriptions of the corneal pathology would seem to be compatible with exposure keratitis and secondary infection resulting from the involvement of the lids that is always present in this variant.

Pemphigoid

In the literature a number of conflicting opinions are expressed concerning the frequency of ocular and other mucosal involvement by pemphigold in its various clinical forms. Recent work suggests that mucous membrane involvement also occurs in other subepidermal bullous dermatoses such as linear IgA disease and chronic bullous disease of childhood. The ocular manifestations of all these are identical and comprise conjunctival ulceration with subsequent healing, fibrosis and scarring to produce the changes of cicatrizing conjunctivitis. The frequency with which skin and one or more mucous membranes is involved seems to vary, but careful examination of the eyes of patients with oral lesions of benign mucous membrane pemphigoid (BMMP) and linear IgA disease (LAD) has shown a high incidence of cicatrizing conjunctival changes in the absence of ocular symptoms.

In its most advanced form the cicatrizing changes of the conjunctiva are easily recognized because the lids become fused to the eyeball, which becomes dry, keratinized and sightless (Figure 2.11). Such late-stage disease is untreatable and it is highly desirable that conjunctival changes are detected as early as possible. The conjunctival changes develop in two ways, either as acute ulcerative lesions or as a quiet cicatrizing process. The former is usually symptom-producing, the

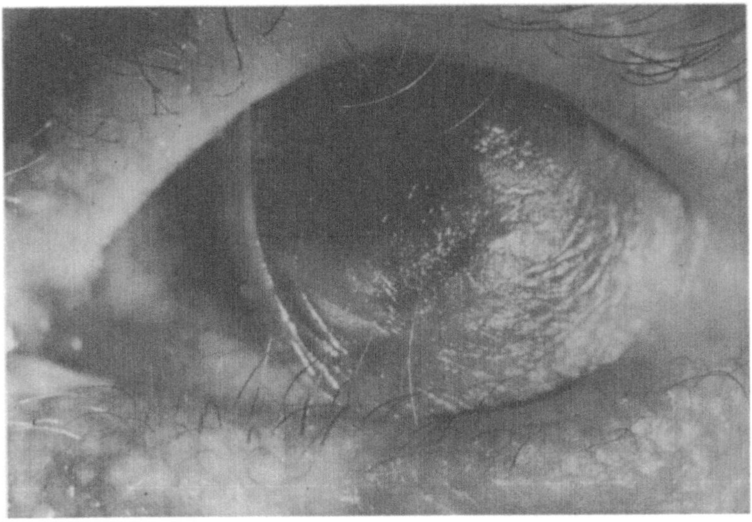

FIGURE 2.11 Advanced ocular cicatricial pemphigoid (OCP)

latter almost always asymptomatic until far advanced. Acute ulcerative lesions present as red eyes with mucoid discharge. The conjunctival ulceration may be difficult to detect without the use of fluorescein, which stains the affected area (Figure 2.12).

The ulceration may occur on any part of the palpebral or bulbar conjunctiva but tends to favour the outer parts of the fornices. The acute ulcerative lesions respond rapidly to intensive topical steroid therapy and then heal without sequelae. If they are not treated, healing occurs slowly over many months and dense localized adhesions between lid and globe occur in the area of the original ulceration. Subsequent ulceration occurs adjacent to the original scarred area and heals with further fibrosis that slowly extends along the length of the fornix to produce shallowing and lid/globe adhesion that can easily be seen with the naked eye. Other patients seem never to have any acute symptomatic episodes but suffer a quiet inflammation of the conjunctiva associated with fibrovascular proliferation. This produces a gradual shrinkage of the conjunctiva that may be harder to detect without specialist examination. The earliest signs are found in the inner canthal regions of the conjunctival sac. In the normal eye there are prominent bumps of tissue and folds of conjunctiva in this region.

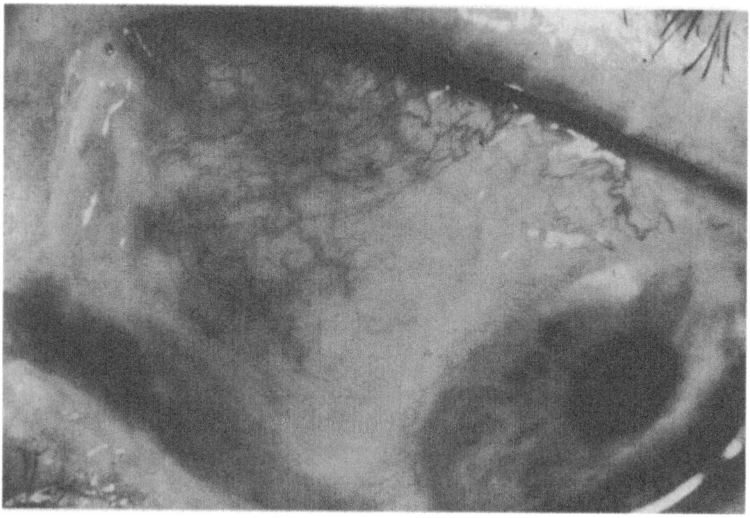

FIGURE 2.12 Active disease with conjunctival ulceration in OCP

The diffuse scarring process in BMMP or LAD produces a flattening out of these structures with a loss of the normal inner canthal architecture. Fornix conjunctiva does not so easily reveal early shrinkage since there are usually capacious folds of conjunctiva present, and so shallowing is only noted at a late stage. Tarsal conjunctiva reveals fibrovascular change more readily, but the appearances require a slit lamp and an experienced observer for their interpretation. The quiet cicatrizing form of the process is not so obviously responsive to topical steroid and the process can spontaneously arrest and remain non-progressive in some patients for many years. In others rapid progression to total fornix obliteration and lid adhesion occurs. These advanced stages of the conjunctival scarring are untreatable. The turning in of the lids (entropion) does not respond to surgery, which instead may produce an exacerbation of the inflammation with increased scarring. Inturning of the lashes, however, can be safely dealt with by cryotherapy to destroy the lash follicles without risk of worsening the underlying disease. The scarring of the conjunctiva involves the ductules emerging from the lacrimal gland so that the eye becomes dry and the ocular surface becomes metaplastic with keratinization. These changes respond very poorly to topical therapy and recent work suggests that a hyperproliferation of the conjunctiva may be the underlying pathological process rather than simple dryness. Surgical treatment to divide the lid/globe adhesions, implant conjunctiva or mucous membrane, or transplant corneal tissue invariably fails. Treatment is with oral steroids, immunosuppressive agents and other drugs such as long-acting sulphonamides and dapsone that have been shown to be effective in the treatment of the skin manifestations of this group of diseases. Topical therapy with artificial tears, lubricant ointments and gels gives some symptomatic relief but the patients often describe severe pain in the eyes and lids that is only relieved when the condition becomes inactive.

CONTACT SENSITIVITY

Contact sensitivity of the lids and periorbital skin is no longer as big a problem, since fewer alkaloids such as atropine and eserine are used for long-term treatment. Antibiotics, especially the aminoglycosides, and preservatives in eye drops are now most often responsible. The causative agent is usually easily recognized and formal patch testing is rarely required. Contact-lens solutions have recently been incriminated in an unusual pattern of contact sensitivity or toxicity caused by the preservatives in the solutions, especially thiomersal. The affected patients have been using the contact-lens solutions for periods of about one year before developing ocular irritation, an epithelial keratitis and superficial vascularization of the upper third of the cornea, with inability to wear the contact lens. The conjunctiva and skin of the lids remain normal and free from inflammation. Withdrawal of the contact lenses and all topical medication results in reversal of the corneal changes. It has been reported that these patients showed positive patch testing to thiomersal and the condition attributed to Type IV hypersensitivity. A group of Moorfields patients investigated at the Institute of Dermatology in London showed negative patch tests but reacted within 24 hours to an ocular challenge with N. saline containing 0.05% thiomersal. The exact mechanisms involved remain unclear, but the contact lenses seem to present the antigenic material to the cornea and conjunctiva in an unusual way, allowing primarily corneal changes without lid or conjunctival signs and without evidence of systemic sensitization.

CATARACT

A cataract is an opacity occurring at any stage of life in the crystalline lens of the eye and the term covers a wide range of changes from the finest asymptomatic congenital dots to dense, sub-total opacities that profoundly reduce vision. Lens opacities are common and close association with other disorders is difficult to prove, but the syndromes and related skin conditions listed in Table 2.2 have been reported.

TABLE 2.2 Conditions associated with lens opacity

Atopic dermatitis
Werner's syndrome (scleropoikiloderma)
Rothmund's syndrome (infantile poikiloderma)
Schäfer's syndrome (congenital dyskeratosis)
Congenital ichthyosiform erythroderma
Siemen's syndrome (congenital skin atrophy)
Bloch–Sulzberger syndrome (incontinentia pigmenti)
Ectodermal dysplasias

RETINAL DISORDERS

A vascular retinopathy can recur in association with any systemic disorder that includes vasculitis. A number of skin conditions can therefore have retinopathy associated with them, either with the basic skin disorder or with any associated hypertension. The picture is usually non-specific. Similarly, a pigmentary retinopathy of the retinitis pigmentosa type can be associated with a number of systemic diseases and syndromes. The presence of the retinopathy may be helpful in establishing the nature of the syndrome, but the appearances are normally those of retinitis pigmentosa.

Angioid streaks

These consist of a bizarre network of reddish-brown striations that appear to lie between the neural retina and the choroid when viewed with the ophthalmoscope. They are usually present bilaterally but are often not symmetrical and they are seen equally in men and women. Advanced examples show a complete ring around the disc with offshoots extending toward the equator of the eye in a radial fashion. The striations are flat with irregular edges and wider than the retinal veins. No branches occur and the appearances are said to resemble cracks in dry mud (Figure 2.13).

Angioid streaks are seen in association with the following conditions:

- Grönblad–Stranberg syndrome (pseudoxanthoma elasticum)
- Ehlers–Danlos syndrome (fibrodysplasia hyperelastica)
- Sickle cell anaemia
- Paget's disease
- Acromegaly
- Lead poisoning

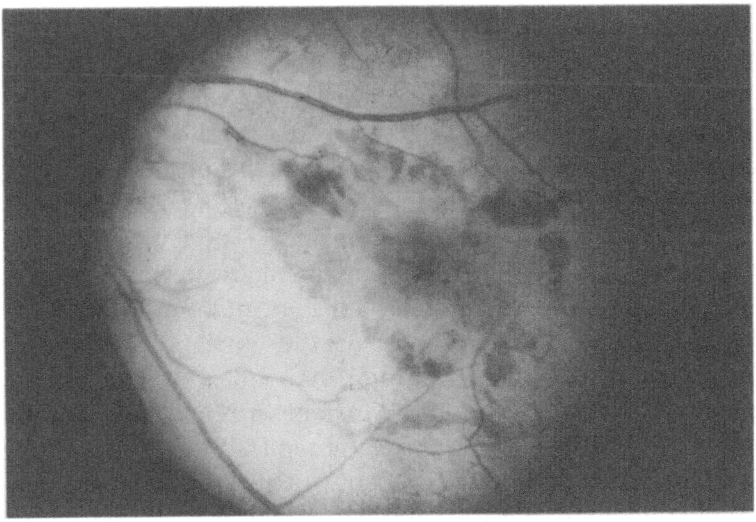

FIGURE 2.13 Angioid streaks with macular haemorrhage

The appearances are thought to be due to ruptures of Bruch's membrane and may be associated with a vascular retinopathy if there is any concomitant hypertension. The ocular changes are asymptomatic in the early stages, but disciform macular degeneration commonly ensues and may result in profound impairment of central vision. No treatment is indicated for the angioid streaks, but laser treatment may be of value in treatment of the early stages of any disciform macular change that may develop.

OCULAR SIDE-EFFECTS OF SKIN TREATMENT

Steroids

Topical steroid applied to lids and periorbital skin can cause dermal atrophy as elsewhere, with increased redness of the lid margins. Whitening of the eye lashes (poliosis) can also occur. Steroid-induced glaucoma and steroid cataract are the main visually damaging complications. Systemic steroids rarely cause glaucoma but may increase previously high/normal intraocular pressures (ocular hypertension) and the risk is greater in offspring of glaucoma sufferers with both systemic and topical steroids. Topical steroids increase the intraocular pressure in 10% of normal individuals and the proportion rises to 30% for glaucoma siblings. Steroid cataract can follow prolonged topical steroid use but most often results from oral administration for a prolonged time. A minimum dose of prednisone 20 mg per day is said to be required over many months. Co-factors such as uveitis or connective tissue disease may be implicated. The typical steroid cataract is posteriorly placed in the lens in the posterior sub-capsular region. The opacity is associated with light diffraction on slit lamp examination to produce a polychromatic appearance that is very similar to the cataract found in atopic individuals.

Steroid cataract once induced can remain remarkably static and non-progressive if systemic steroids are reduced or replaced by other forms of treatment. However, because of its locations, the opacity causes maximum visual disturbance especially in bright light or under conditions of glare such as night driving, so that early surgical treatment is usually indicated.

Psoralen/UVA (PUVA) therapy[10,11]

The development of this form of treatment has occurred at a time when concern has been growing about ocular phototoxicity, and a number of studies have shown that the retinal damage threshold occurs at wavelengths in the blue region of the spectrum. Normally this potential hazard is offset by the progressive development of yellow pigmentation of the adult lens to create a very effective UV filter. Apart from the possible direct hazard of UV radiation on ocular tissues there is also a greatly enhanced risk from photosensitized reactions in the lens, because from an early stage of development the ocular lens is completely encapsulated by epithelium and so accumulates cells throughout its life. Photobinding of any compound to the lens constituents therefore ensures lifelong retention within the lens and a unique potential for damage by photosensitization. The psoralens, especially 8-methoxypsoralen (8-MOP) used in PUVA therapy for the treatment of skin disorders including psoriasis and vitiligo, have been shown to be present in ocular tissues within 2 hours of a single dose and can become photobound to this protein and DNA if there is concurrent exposure to ambient levels of UVA radiation. The adult ocular lens as previously described acts as an efficient filter so there is no photobinding to retina in normal eyes, but this tissue is at risk in patients following cataract surgery or in young eyes when the lens still permits significant passage of UVA. Modern intra-ocular lenses inserted after cataract surgery incorporate UVA barrier compounds. Psoralen/UVA therapy and cataract formation has been documented in experimental animals and clinically observed human cataracts have been reported. Cataracts from patients who received PUVA therapy have been examined in detail, and the lens proteins show phosphorescence peaks identical to the 8-MOP protein photoproducts seen in experimental animals. Fortunately, 8-MOP can only be found in the lens for 24 hours after ingestion, provided that the eye is protected from UVA radiation. Patients should therefore be provided with appropriate UV filtering glasses to be worn from the time of ingestion of the drug and for the following 24 hours, indoors as well as outdoors since there is sufficient UVA in ordinary fluorescent lighting to photobind the 8-MOP. Objective methods of studying fluorescence in human lenses in the living eye have shown that with these precautions patients receiving PUVA show no enhanced fluorescence, while a control group treated prior to recognition of the need for ocular protection showed anomalous, enhanced fluorescence and clinical cataract formation. It is of interest that patients on long-term penicillamine treatment show lower than normal levels of lens fluorescence because penicillamine acts as a free-radical scavenger and chelating agent to prevent lens damage from insults, including photodamage.

Chloroquine and other antimalarials[12–15]

This group of drugs has been used for treatment of connective tissue diseases and photodermatoses for many years. Initial enthusiasm for their use was diminished by the reports of irreversible ocular damage with profound visual loss caused by chloroquine and hydroxychloroquine, but a new vogue for their use seems to have occurred. The same eye complications have been recorded after long-term use of both hydroxychloroquine and chloroquine, so the two drugs will be discussed as one, although hydroxychloroquine appears safer.

The ocular adverse reaction to chloroquine is dose and time related, but no clear limits for total dosage have emerged and duration of treatment prior to onset of symptoms or signs has varied from 7 months to 10 years. A total dose of 100 g (a little over 200 mg per day for a year) of chloroquine base seems to be a useful upper safe limit, or a daily dose of less than 6.5 mg/kg of hydroxychloroquine. The drug is retained for very long periods in the body and in the eye as a result of binding to melanin. Direct damage also occurs to the ganglion cells of the retina. Drug excretion in the urine has been shown 5 years after treatment was discontinued and attempts to increase excretion or displace bound drug have not been successful. The ocular findings are corneal deposition and a toxic retinopathy. The reported incidence of retinal complications varies from 0 to 22% and the incidence of corneal complications from 30 to 70%. Recent work has suggested that hydroxychloroquine may cause fewer eye complications than chloroquine and no complications were seen in 900 patients if the daily dose was kept below 6.5 mg/kg. In the cornea the deposits, possibly chloroquine itself, are found within the phagosomes of the basal cells of the corneal epithelium. The intra-phagosomal material renders the cells opaque, yellowish-brown in colour, and they can be seen forming a swirled pattern (cornea verticillata) across the lower third of the cornea on slit lamp examination. Early stages of deposition are difficult to detect and even the most advanced changes cannot be seen with the naked eye or ophthalmoscope. The intra-epithelial deposits rarely cause any symptoms and, although heavy deposition may cause the patient to see haloes around bright light sources, they appear benign and disappear completely within 6 weeks of discontinuing drug treatment. The retinal damage, on the other hand, does not reverse and may progress to blindness or profound visual loss even after the drug is discontinued. The retinal lesions comprise an initial oedema and ring pigmentary change around the macula to cause a bulls-eye or doughnut-like appearance that progresses to a widespread pigmentary retinal degeneration with narrowed retinal vessels and secondary optic atrophy.

Monitoring of patients on long-term chloroquine treatment is mandatory but presents a number of problems. Early intra-corneal deposition may not be easy to detect even on slit lamp examination, and although corneal changes usually precede retinal damage this is not invariable. Retinal changes need to be monitored every 3–6 months whilst the patient remains on treatment and a pre-treatment fundus examination is essential because considerable individual variation in macular pigmentation occurs and may make the detection of early changes very difficult. Visual acuity and visual fields to a red target are useful tests. The central field to red can easily be tested using the red grid pattern of the standard Amslers charts. Electrophysiological responses of the retinal cells should in theory provide the most sensitive tests for retinal toxicity, but the results appear conflicting in published reports, the tests are time-consuming and not widely available.

Mepacrine can produce yellow discolouration of conjunctiva and cornea that is asymptomatic, and the drug has rarely been associated with an optic neuritis.

REFERENCES

1. McCulley, J. P., Dougherty, J. M. and Deneau, D. G. (1982). Classification of chronic blepharitis. *Ophthalmology (Rochester)*, **89,** 1173–80
2. Dougherty, J. M. and McCulley, J. P. (1986). Bacterial lipases and chronic blepharitis. *Invest. Ophthalmol. Vis. Sci.*, **27,** 486–91
3. McCulley, J. P. and Dougherty, J. M. (1985). Blepharitis associated with acne rosacea and seborrhoeic dermatitis. In Callen, J. P. and Eifferman, R. A. (eds.) *International Ophthalmology Clinics (Oculocutaneous Diseases)* Vol. 25, No. 1 pp. 159–72 (Boston: Little, Brown & Co.)
4. McCulley, J. P. and Sciallis, G. F. (1983). Meibomian keratoconjunctivitis: oculodermal correlates. *Contact Intraocul. Lens Med. J.*, **9,** 130–2
5. Jenkins, M. S., Brown, S. I., Lempert, S. L. and Weinberg, R. J. (1979). Ocular rosacea. *Am. J. Ophthalmol.*, **88,** 618–22
6. Leonard, J. N., Wright, P., Williams, D. M., Gilkes, J. J. H., Haffenden, G. P., McMinn, R. M. H. and Fry, L. (1984). The relationship between linear IgA disease and benign mucous membrane pemphigoid. *Br. J. Dermatol.*, **110,** 307–14
7. Marsden, R. A. and Greaves, M. W. (1983). Atypical bullous dermatosis of childhood with entropion. *J. R. Soc. Med.*, **75,** 908
8. Wojnarowska, F., Marsden, R. A., Bhogal, B. and Black, M. M. (1984). Childhood cicatricial pemphigoid with linear IgA deposits. *Clin. Exp. Dermatol.*, **9,** 407–15
9. Wright, P. (1986). Cicatrizing conjunctivitis. *Trans. Ophthalmol. Soc. UK*, **105,** 1–17
10. Stern, R. S., Parrish, J. A. and Fitzpatrick, T. B. (1985). Ocular findings in patients treated with P.U.V.A. *J. Invest. Dermatol.*, **85,** 269–73
11. Lerman, S. (1985). Ocular phototoxicity. In Davidson, S. I. and Frauenfelder, F. T. (eds) *Recent Advances in Ophthalmology*, pp. 109–36. Edinburgh: Churchill Livingstone
12. Mantyjarvi, M. (1985). Hydroxychloroquine treatment and the eye. *Scand. J. Rheumatol.*, **14,** 171–4
13. Tobin, D. R., Krohel, G. B. and Rynes, R. I. (1982). Hydroxychloroquine, seven years experience. *Arch. Ophthalmol.*, **100,** 81–3
14. Finbloom, D. S., Silver, K., Newsome, D. A. and Gunkel, R. (1985). Comparison of hydroxychloroquine and chloroquine use and the development of retinal toxicity. *J. Rheumatol.*, **12** (4), 692–4
15. Mackenzie, A. H. (1983). Dose refinements in long term therapy of rheumatoid arthritis with antimalarials. *Am. J. Med.*, **75,** 40–3

3

SARCOIDOSIS AND THE SKIN

C. M. E. ROWLAND PAYNE

INTRODUCTION

Sarcoidosis is an idiopathic systemic granulomatous disorder with a predilection for the reticulo-endothelial system, lungs, eyes and skin[1–6]. Clinical signs vary greatly and depend on the immunological state and race of the patient, the age and activity of the disease and the anatomical site of involvement. Cutaneous manifestations occur in up to half of patients[7] and vary greatly.

The disease is commonest in West Indians and Irish populations[7] and preferentially affects females aged less than 40[1]. The prognosis is best in young Irish females[7].

Two patterns of cutaneous involvement can be distinguished: the microscopically granulomatous and the simply reactive such as erythema nodosum. Neither pattern is unequivocally diagnostic but, in most cases, after a detailed history and physical examination, the diagnosis can be made on clinical grounds and quickly confirmed by lesional biopsy.

Skin lesions give an indication of the age, activity and prognosis of the disease. Their observation or serial biopsy can be used to monitor disease activity and response to treatment. It was as a skin disease that sarcoidosis was first recorded[8].

Perhaps more than any other disease, sarcoidosis illustrates that dermatology is an essential part of general medicine. The appearance of a few cutaneous lesions may explain a previously undiagnosable succession of minor complaints and ill health, such as dry eyes, a Bell's palsy and the finding of raised liver enzyme values.

REACTIVE LESIONS

Erythema nodosum (EN)

EN[9] is the commonest cutaneous manifestation of sarcoidosis. It occurs in up to 30% of patients[7] and is frequently the presenting feature of the disease.

EN is common in White Britons, especially Celts and those with the HLA B8 phenotype[10], and is rare in Blacks and Orientals[10]. In the North London series of 818 mainly White patients[7], 30% (251) had EN, whereas in the Washington DC series of 127 Black patients[11] only 2% (3) had EN. EN is a good prognostic sign. Of the North London series, 84% of those with EN were in remission within 2 years[7]. In the same series, only 15% of those with lupus pernio were in remission after 2 years[7].

EN represents a non-specific reaction pattern. Circulating immune complexes probably lodge in the slow-flowing and cooler vessels of the subcutaneous fat, where they cause a focal septal panniculitis[12] (Figure 3.1). This inflammation principally affects the fibrous septa between the lobules of the subcutaneous fat. The microscopic appearances vary with the age of the lesion. Initially the septa become widened by extravasation of oedema fluid, lymphocytes and some polymorphonuclear leukocytes, and later by red cells. Soon the inflammatory changes spill out of the septa into the lobules. In the second week lymphocytes and histiocytes predominate, with occasional giant cells but without granuloma formation. Finally there is complete resolution. Throughout its course the septal vessel walls remain relatively unharmed and there is no true vasculitis. Because EN is a focal inflammation, incisional biopsy must be generous and include the full thickness of the subcutaneous fat, down as far as the deep fascia. No histological features distinguish EN attributable to sarcoidosis from EN due to other causes.

Clinically, there is a transient symmetrical eruption with a predilection for the anterior shins of young women (Figure 3.2). Lesions pass through all the changes associated with the resolution of a bruise.

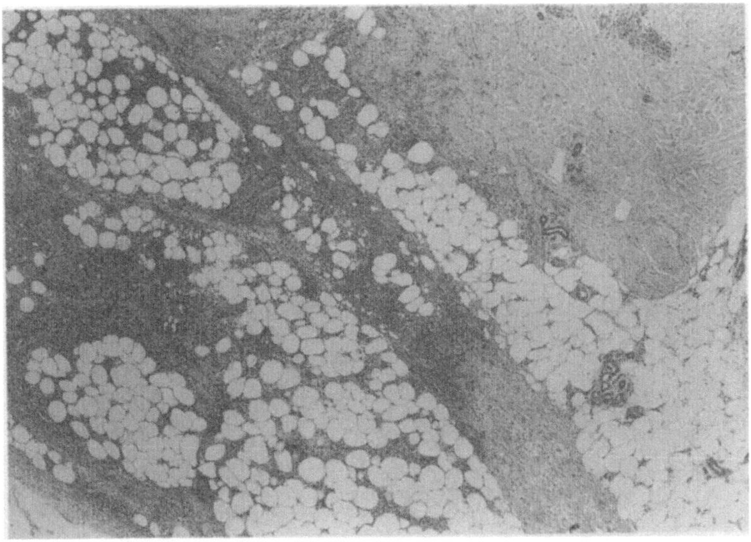

FIGURE 3.1 *Erythema nodosum* is a septal panniculitis (H&E × 30)

At first tender and erythematous, within days a subcutaneous nodule forms that becomes raised up and somewhat purpuric with a violaceous colour that gives way, over a period of weeks, to shades of brown and green, finally resolving without scarring. Sometimes lesions are more widespread, involving the upper limbs and abdomen, but they are always most numerous on the extensor aspects of the dependent parts.

Up to half of those with EN have Löfgren's syndrome[13], in which the skin lesions are associated with fever, lymphadenopathy and arthralgia, particularly affecting the ankle joints.

GRANULOMATOUS LESIONS

The granuloma is essentially a natural defence mechanism the purpose of which is to entrap and neutralize foreign material, especially infective foreign material. Its pathophysiological acme is illustrated by the calcified 'apical' lung tuberculous granuloma that is sometimes detected by chest radiograph as an incidental finding in fit patients.

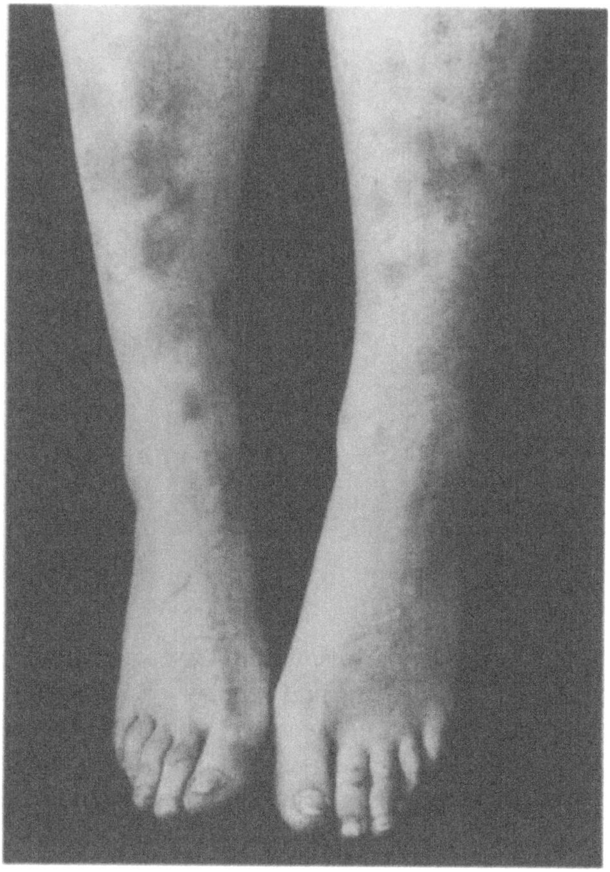

FIGURE 3.2 *Erythema nodosum* favours the anterior shins

Granulomatous infiltration is a form of inflammation characterized by bundles of macrophages. When macrophages (syn: histiocytes, epithelioid cells) clump together they are known as granulomas (syn: sarcoids, tubercles). The course of granulomatous infiltration is much slower than that of EN. Although granulomatous infiltration has many causes, certain microscopic features hint at a particular aetiology.

In sarcoidosis (Figure 3.3) scattered, neatly formed granulomas are made up of dense clusters of macrophages which, in places, coalesce to form Langhan's multinucleate giant cells. Around the granulomas

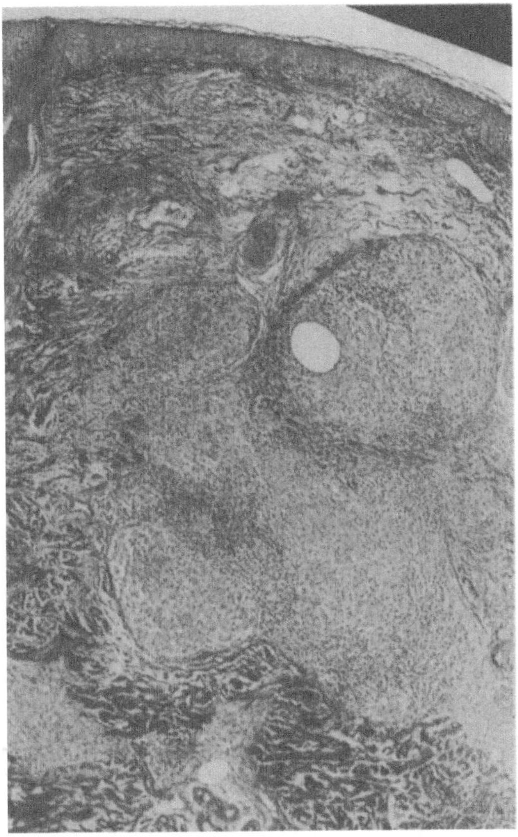

FIGURE 3.3 *Sarcoidosis.* The upper dermis is filled with neatly circumscribed granulomas (Picro-Mallory × 40)

the lymphocytic infiltrate is sparse ('naked granulomas'). Caseation does not occur. As the process ages, the granulomas are replaced by fibrous tissue. At any moment all the lesions appear to be of the same age and the overall impression is well-ordered and tidy, in contrast with lupus vulgaris (Figure 3.4).

Sarcoidal granulomas can occur in any organ and at any site within an organ. They can be single or scattered or multiple and coalescing. They evolve with time from small collections of macrophages to large, tightly bundled granulomas that are finally replaced by fibrous scar

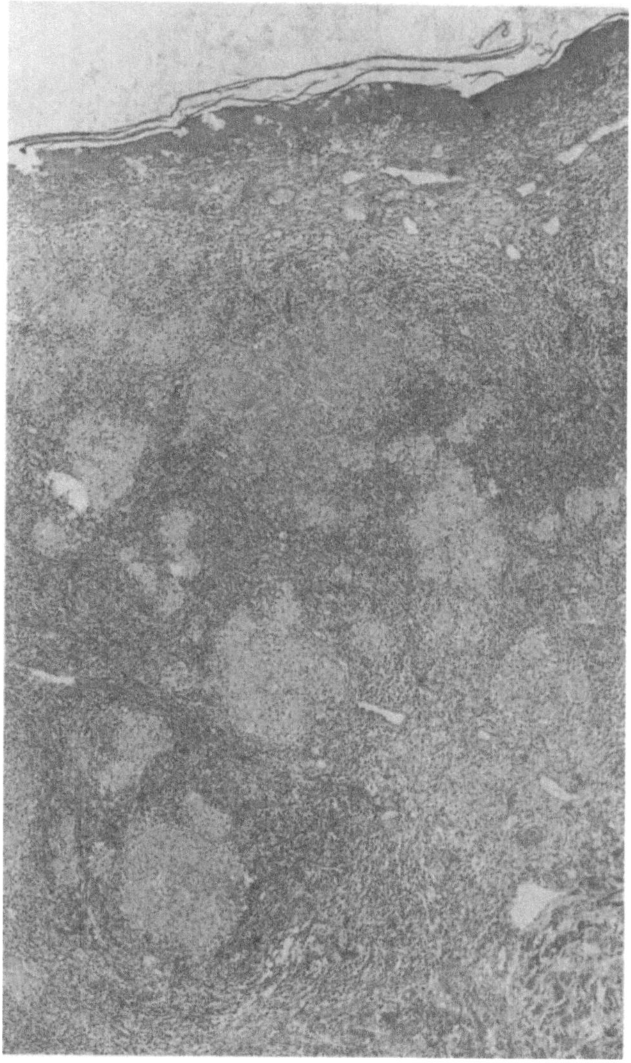

FIGURE 3.4 *Lupus vulgaris*. In tuberculosis of the skin granulomas affect the upper dermis but they are less tidy and more destructive than in sarcoidosis (Picro-Mallory × 40)

tissue, sometimes even resolving completely. With such variability of disease expression, it is almost surprising that there is ever a classical dermatological appearance of sarcoidosis.

Granulomatous skin lesions affect about 10–20% of patients[10], and they are commoner and more diverse in Blacks. Usually they are manifest as papules, nodules and plaques.

Papules

Papules have a predilection for the face, especially the beard area and perioral skin. Typically, they are symmetrical, numerous and scattered uniformly over the affected area. They begin as pinkish, erythematous, lentil-sized elements that soon become more brownish and waxy. Apart from a minimal degree of surface scaling, the epidermis is largely unaffected. As time passes, the lesions spread outward, becoming *annular*, leaving hyper- or hypo-pigmented, slightly scarred centres. In Blacks, the pigmentary changes are strikingly obvious. Diascopy (pressure with a watch glass), drives the blood from the lesions, revealing the characteristic yellowish opalescent 'lupoid grains' corresponding to the dermal conglomerates of the microscopic granulomas.

True *micropapular sarcoidosis*[14] is an almost exanthematic eruption affecting the trunk, particularly the periumbilical skin and upper back (Figure 3.5). The lesions are usually symptomless and comprise confluent sheets of countless erythematous macules and erythematous, slightly yellowish-brown, almost translucent, pinhead-sized papules. In due course the lesions disappear without scarring. This syndrome probably indicates a highly active granulomatous phase of the disease. *Lichenoid sarcoidosis* is probably a variant of this.

Nodules

Papules and nodules differ only in size. As more granulomas collect, a lesion may move from one category to the next. Nodules are characteristically smooth and purplish swellings over which the epidermis is stretched. Nodules that are more vascular and have an orangish

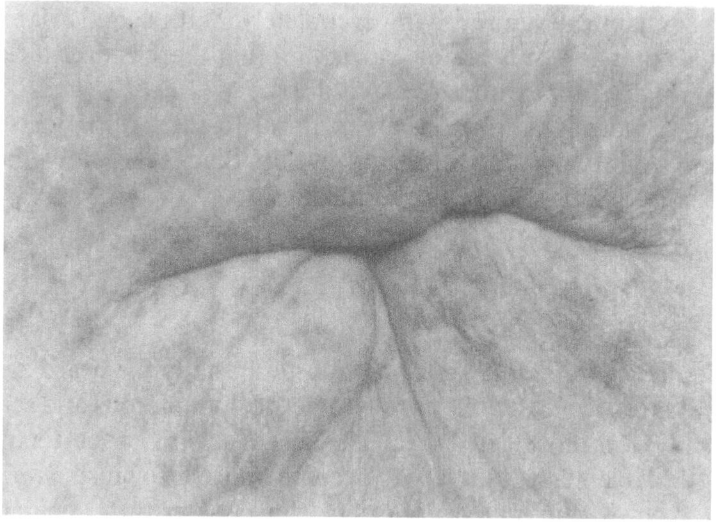

FIGURE 3.5 *Micropapular sarcoidosis* favours the trunk

colour, with vessels coursing over their surface, are known as *angiolupoid nodules* and are most often seen on the side of a female patient's nose.

Darier-Roussy sarcoids (syn: subcutaneous sarcoidosis) are an uncommon and characteristically asymptomatic form of nodular sarcoidosis in which there is a granulomatous panniculitis. Half a dozen walnut-sized, painless, cold and fluctuant, untethered, subcutaneous nodules are found scattered over the limbs. They last months or years and, in general, eventually resolve spontaneously. In rare cases they ulcerate (Figure 3.6)[15].

Scar sarcoidosis results from granulomatous infiltration of existing scars. This Köbnerization may affect recent or long-standing scars (Figure 3.7). It usually occurs early in the course of the disease and may herald the onset of uveitis[4]. Scar sarcoidosis may occur at the sites of operations, tuberculin tests[4], venepuncture, ear-piercing[16], tattoos and other scars. Indeed, the development of a foreign body granuloma in an old scar may occasionally be the first sign of sarcoidosis[17].

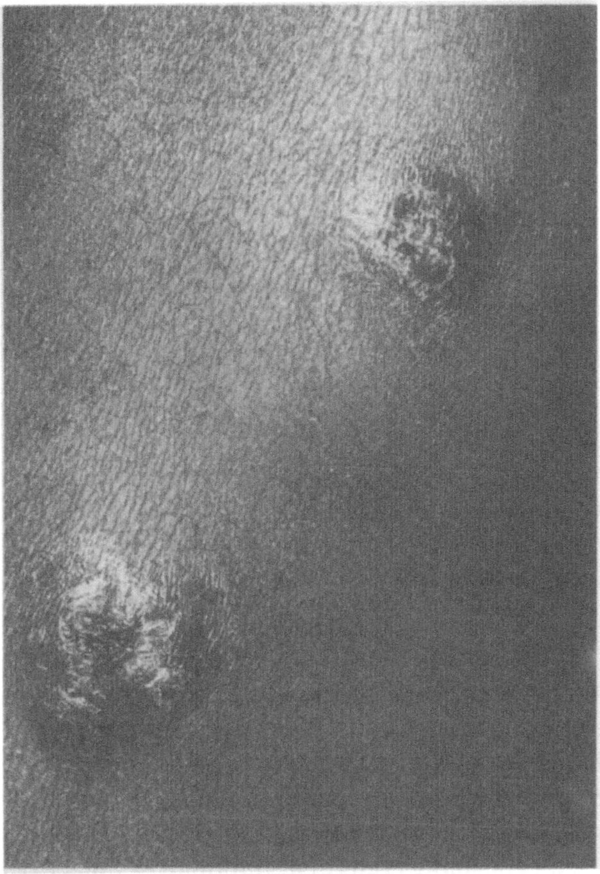

FIGURE 3.6 *Ulcerative Darier–Roussy sarcoids.* Walnut-sized subcutaneous granulomatous abscesses may ulcerate

Plaques

Plaque sarcoids are raised patches formed from coalescing or outwardly spreading papules. Papules, nodules and plaques simply represent increasingly larger aggregates of granulomas with a correspondingly poorer prognosis.

Lupus pernio[8] is the commonest form of plaque sarcoidosis[18]. The plaques have an affinity for the colder parts of the body, such as the tip of the nose (Figure 3.8), the cheeks (where the fat pads insulate

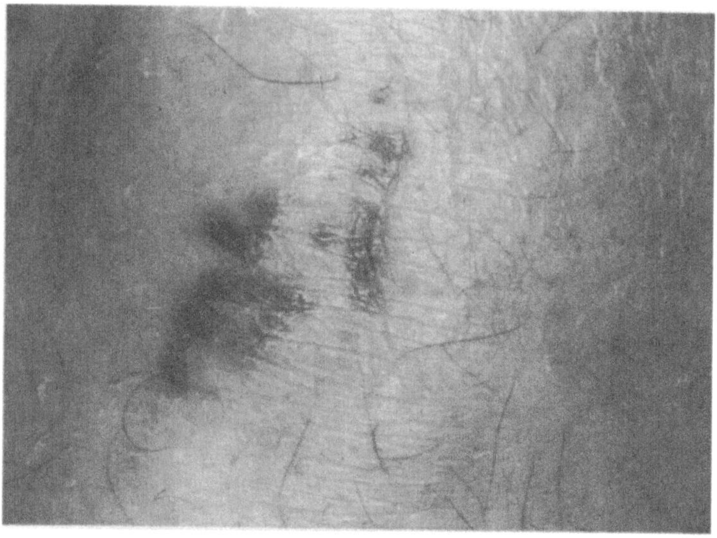

Figure 3.7 *Scar sarcoidosis.* Sarcoidal granulomas may affect new or long-standing scars

the skin from the warmth of the muscular blood supply), the lobes of the ears, the tips of the toes and the dorsa of the fingers. The lesions are purplish and swollen with ill-defined edges. They are cold and firm to the touch and their surface is often scaly and may easily become eroded. In patients with lupus pernio, the mucous membranes of nose and upper airways usually contain granulomas. Lupus pernio is more common in older women, especially West Indians, and is commonly associated with hypercalcaemia and with chronic fibrotic sarcoidosis affecting other organs, especially the upper respiratory tract and bones[5,18]. Three quarters of West Indian women with lupus pernio have intrathoracic sarcoidosis[18].

Kviem–Siltzbach test

Material derived from homogenized sarcoidal spleen provokes a granulomatous response in most patients with active sarcoidosis. It has a false positive rate of less than 2% and is sensitive enough to have been positive in 78% of 2189 patients[19]. It is especially helpful

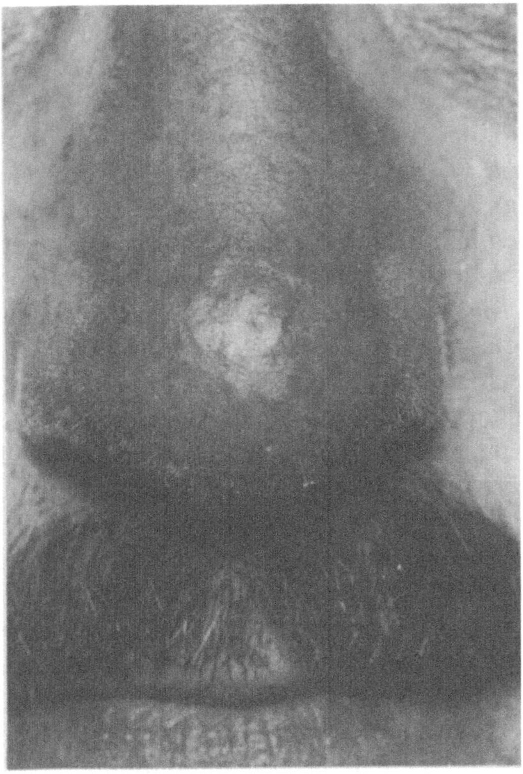

Figure 3.8 *Lupus pernio*. Early lesions favour the cold extremities, such as the tip of the nose

in active sarcoidosis. It may often be negative in fibrotic burnt-out disease. The same is true of the serum angiotensin-converting enzyme level, which may be regarded as the erythrocyte sedimentation rate of granulomatous inflammation.

UNUSUAL CUTANEOUS MANIFESTATIONS OF SARCOIDOSIS

Cutaneous sarcoidosis is a disease of signs rather than symptoms. *Pain* is most exceptional and in one patient it was brought on by alcohol and hot showers[20]. *Pruritus* of cutaneous granulomas is most unusual[21]. *Generalized pruritus* is usually associated with deranged liver function due to granulomatous hepatitis[22], but presumably may also result from hypercalcaemia of sarcoidosis. *Prurigo*[6], an intensely pruritic eruption characterized by marked excoriations, and even *nodular prurigo*[23] may occur. Sometimes larger plaques of lichenification[21] may develop, or *verrucous plaques*[24], mimicking tuberculosis or deep mycotic infections. The more unusual, severe and *fulminant forms* of sarcoidosis are predominantly a problem of the Black races[5].

Facial oedema[25] is rare. Resolution of large facial lesions may leave pendulous folds of *chalazoderma*[6] imitating cutis laxa. Granulomas in the lid lymphatics may cause eyelid swelling, unilateral eyelid oedema and even unilateral proptosis. *Conjunctival granulomas* occur in up to one third of patients[26] and may be useful diagnostically. Unusually, a *sicca syndrome*[4] may develop with keratoconjunctivitis sicca, xerostomia and salivary gland enlargement requiring differentiation from Sjögren's syndrome. *Nasal stuffiness*[27] with 'winter hay fever', intranasal brown crusts, purulent mucus and widening of the bridge of the nose is not uncommon in sarcoidosis. These features indicate involvement of the nasal mucosa and bone. Nasal mucosal biopsy is simple and helpful. Nasal cartilage can be destroyed by the disease, leading to perforation of the septum. *Mucosal granulomas* also occur in the buccal mucosa, palate, larynx and tongue.

Granulomatous alopecia[28–30] is not only manifest on the scalp[28,29], where it may be cicatricial[31] or patchy, but may also affect the limbs[30]. *Follicular papules*[32] may be spinous and are more common in childhood than in adult life. *Perifollicular pustules and papules* scattered over the body have been reported[3].

True histologically confirmed *erythema multiforme*[33] has been reported as the presenting feature of sarcoidosis and *erythema multiforme-like* lesions[34] that are histologically granulomatous may also occur. *Granulomatous vasculitis*[35] can, on the head and neck, simulate erythema annulare centrifugum, granuloma faciale and Sweet's disease. Sarcoidosis can cause *thrombophlebitis*[36] of the limbs (Figure 3.9) and *capillaritis*.

Upper dermal granulomatous inflammation may cause some overlying desquamation, *granulomatous ichthyosis*[37]. Less pronounced inflammation can cause *hypopigmented sarcoidosis*[38,39] (Figure 3.10) which typically affects Black females in the third or fourth decade and

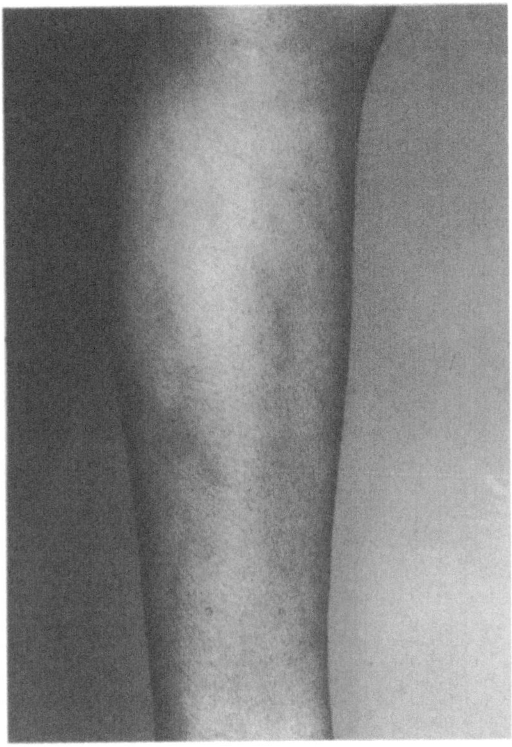

Figure 3.9 *Sarcoidal thrombophlebitis.* Rarely, sarcoidal inflammation affects blood vessels

often affects the extremities. Granulomas lie beneath the hypopigmented macules and leprosy must be excluded. The limbs are also affected by *nummular eczema-like* lesions[40], *atrophy*[41] and *anetoderma*[41].

Ulceration, though not a typical feature of sarcoidosis, does occur, notably leg ulceration[15,42]. It complicates pre-existing granulomatous lesions such as plaques or psoriasiform lesions[43], especially those that are atrophic or cicatricial. *Elephantine sarcoidosis*[44], in which there is often asymmetrical pseudolymphoedema, is also prone to ulceration. Ulceration of subcutaneous sarcoidosis is not unusual[15]. In the very rare '*formes sphacéliques*'[6] the patient is febrile and the nodules are painful, break down, and become gangrenous.

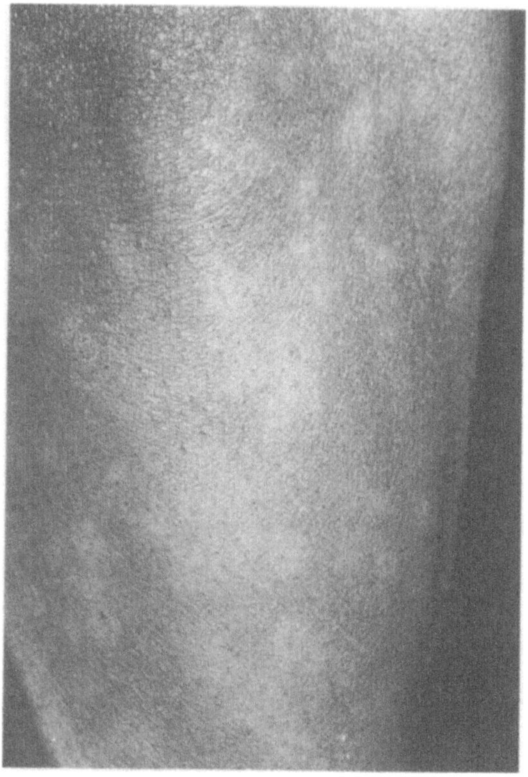

Figure 3.10 *Hypopigmented sarcoidosis* should be distinguished from leprosy

Palmoplantar sarcoidosis[31] may be erythemato-squamous and somewhat suggestive of secondary syphilis or more keratotic and psoriasiform[3]. *Dactylitis* and digital oedema occur[25]. Like the sausage fingers of dactylitis, *nail sarcoidosis*[45,46] is frequently associated with lupus pernio of the digits and underlying osseous sarcoidosis. The nail plate may become pitted, cracked, brittle and dystrophic, longitudinally ridged, thickened, clubbed, fragile and eventually lost. Pterygium formation may occur, simulating lichen planus. In nail sarcoidosis granulomas are found in the nail bed.

An acute *eruptive form of sarcoidosis* (which may be the same as the so-called 'erythrodermic sarcoidosis') occurs in which, over a matter of weeks, a roughly symmetrical eruption develops that favours the limbs and is characterized by brightly erythematous papules and plaques, often with a scaly surface. Lesions of all ages are present from new, firm erythematous papules to rather browner elements with depressed centres. Histology may be misleading as giant cells may be absent from the early lesions. A true generalized erythroderma or exfoliative dermatitis due to sarcoidosis is unknown. *Vulval and peri-anal sarcoidosis*[47] are rare sites for the papular form of sarcoidosis. Sarcoidosis may occur in an *actinic*[48] distribution and the clinical presentation may mimic polymorphic light eruption. *Aestival sarcoidosis*[49] recurs each spring and resolves each autumn. It too has an actinic component. *Calcinosis cutis*[40] probably represents the ultimate sequel of fibrotic granulomas.

DEBATABLE AREAS

There are some debatable areas of histological differential diagnosis. *Necrobiosis lipoidica* (NL) usually affects the anterior shins. In NL streaks of deep dermal degeneration of collagen are surrounded by a sparse histiocytic infiltrate; giant cells are unusual. Sometimes there is real difficulty in distinguishing between NL and sarcoidosis[50]. When NL occurs on the head, *atypical facial necrobiosis of Dowling and Wilson Jones*[50] (Figure 3.11), the histological appearances are even closer to sarcoidosis than when necrobiosis occurs at other sites. *Granuloma annulare* (GA) is a pathological process similar to NL but occurring more superficially in the dermis, and the clinical signs are seen not on the shins but on the hands and feet or wrists and ankles (Figure 3.12). *Actinic granuloma of O'Brien* is the appearance of GA in an actinic distribution[51].

NL and GA are idiopathic granulomatous cutaneous eruptions. Each may occur as an isolated transient phenomenon in otherwise healthy patients. Each is more common in patients with diabetes mellitus (types 1 and 11)[52,53]. Sometimes NL and GA occur in the same patient[52]. Of all these debatable areas the differential diagnosis of sarcoidosis, NL and GA is perhaps the most difficult.

GA has been reported with sarcoidosis[54]. Was the GA an associated disease or a feature of sarcoidosis? Put another way, can sarcoidosis manifest itself in the skin as a GA-like eruption? Similarly, NL and

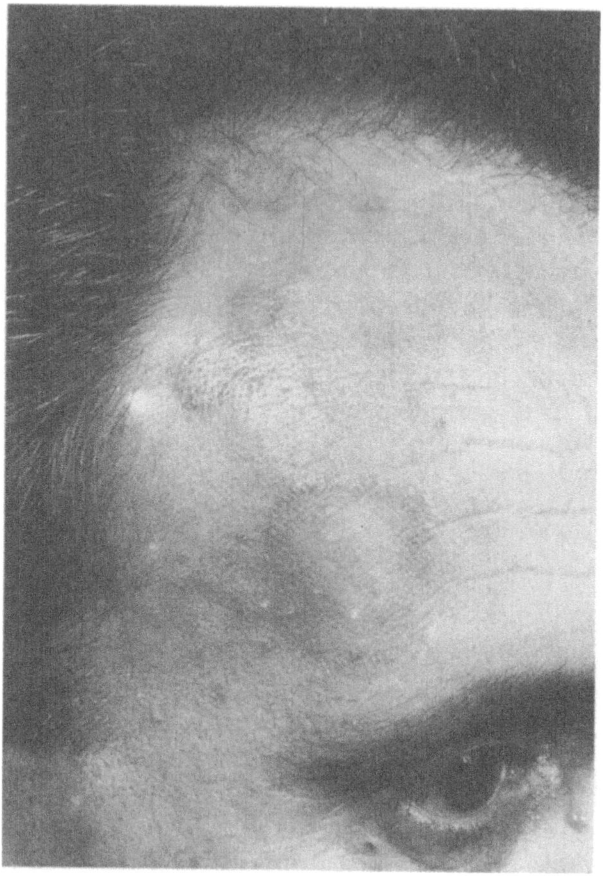

Figure 3.11 *Dowling–Wilson Jones syndrome* has similarities with both sarcoidosis and necrobiosis lipoidica

sarcoidosis sometimes coexist[55,56]. Is this the coexistence of NL and sarcoidosis or have the granulomas of sarcoidosis caused an NL-like eruption? Atypical facial necrobiosis and sarcoidosis can coexist[57]. Surely such occurrences cannot be viewed as chance associations of different diseases. An illustrative patient was recently reported[58]. This woman had systemic sarcoidosis, diabetes and extensive NL. On the legs the NL ulcerated; on the face it caused atrophic annular lesions identical to the atypical necrobiosis of Dowling–Wilson Jones. Seven biopsies from this patient showed how the histology was similar in

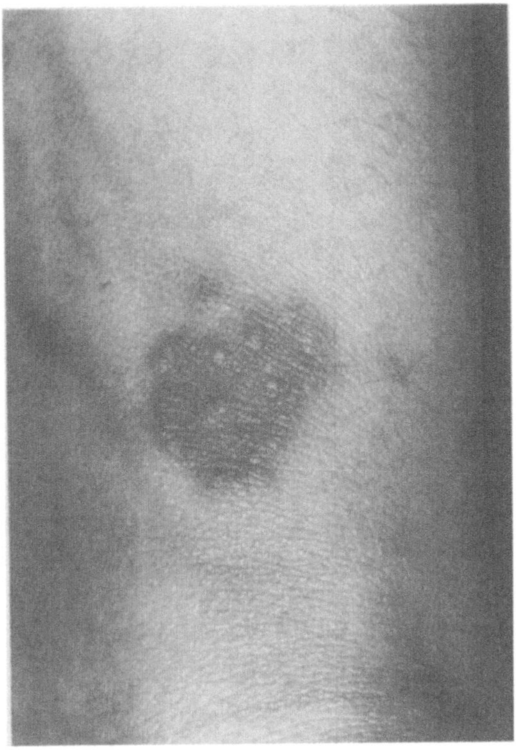

Figure 3.12 *Granuloma annulare* may sometimes coexist with sarcoidosis

all areas. The clinical manifestation of this patient's granulomatous disorder appeared to be modified by the anatomical site. Surely all the lesions were due to the sarcoidosis.

Granulomatous involvement of the skin has been recorded in *Crohn's disease*. In *Miescher's granulomatous cheilitis* (Figure 3.13) (which is histologically indistinguishable from sarcoidosis and may occur in association with Crohn's disease or systemic sarcoid) there is localized lymphoedema that is usually a sequel to recurrent erysipelas. Granulomatous cheilitis is also seen in the *Melkersson–Rosenthal syndrome*, in which a scrotal tongue is associated with recurrent attacks of lip swelling and facial nerve palsy. *Rheumatoid nodules* have a granulomatous histology and have occurred in association with sarcoidosis[59], NL[60] and GA[60]. The histological similarities between these disorders and certain forms of sarcoidosis are striking.

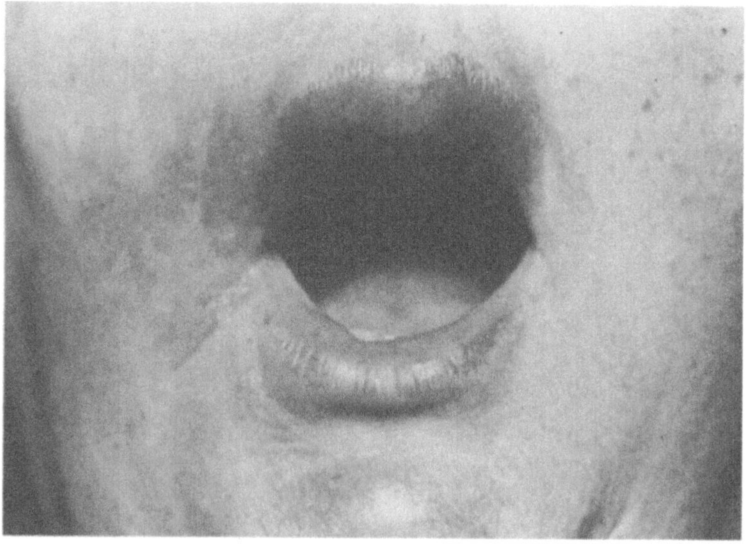

Figure 3.13 *Granulomatous cheilitis* may occur alone or as a manifestation of sarcoidosis or Crohn's disease

Sarcoidosis has been defined as an idiopathic granulomatous disorder affecting two or more organs[4]. However convincing cases of disseminated, though strictly cutaneous, disease have been recorded[61].

The clinical manifestations of sarcoidosis are determined by the host genotype. EN and arthritis occur more readily in those with the HLA B8 phenotype[10]. *Psoriasiform lesions*[43,62] probably represent a psoriatic response (köbnerization) to dermal granulomas. Similarly, lichenified and nodular prurigo-like lesions[23] probably represent an atopic eczematous response to scratching caused, for example, by generalized pruritus itself consequent upon sarcoidal hepatitis.

Finally, should sarcoidosis be viewed as an autoimmune disease? EN, iritis, Sjögren's syndrome and thyroiditis are clinical features shared by sarcoidosis and many autoimmune diseases, as are the laboratory findings of raised gamma globulins, circulating antibodies, defective suppressor T cell function[63] and the phenotype HLA B8 DR3. More impressive are reports of sarcoidosis coexisting with autoimmune thyroid disease[64], Addison's disease[64], autoimmune thrombocytopenia[65] and haemolytic anaemia[65], pernicious anaemia[66] vitiligo[64,66] and lichen sclerosus et atrophicus[66], primary biliary cirrhosis[63] and progressive systemic sclerosis[63]. Are these simply chance associations or do they indicate a common immunological thread?

CONCLUSION

The skin is involved in half of all patients with sarcoidosis. The disease often presents in the skin and its course can be monitored by serial observation of the skin.

The cutaneous lesions of sarcoidosis are visible and readily biopsied. Some lesions, such as EN, are very common and others, such as lupus pernio, are easy to recognize.

The skin is a signpost to the diagnosis of sarcoidosis.

ACKNOWLEDGEMENTS

The author is very grateful to Dr M. M. Black for permission to publish photographs of his patients, to Dr A. C. Branfoot for some of the photomicrographs, to the Medical Illustration departments of St Thomas's, Westminster and St Stephen's Hospitals, London, and to Mrs Kathleen Fowler for help with typing the manuscript.

REFERENCES

1. Cronin, E. (1970). Skin changes in sarcoidosis. *Postgrad. Med. J.*, **46,** 507–9
2. Perroud, A. M., Revuz, J. and Touraine, R. (1983). Sarcoïdose cutanée. *Le Revue du Practicien,* **33,** 2051–60
3. Scadding, J. G. and Mitchell, D. N. (1985). *Sarcoidosis.* (London: Chapman & Hall)
4. James, D. G. and Williams, W. J. (1985). *Sarcoidosis and Other Granulomatous Disorders.* (Philadelphia: Saunders)
5. Savin, J. A. and Wilkinson, D. S. (1986). Sarcoidosis. In Rook, A., Wilkinson, D. S., Ebling, F. J.G., Champion, R. H. and Burton, J. L. (eds.) *Textbook of Dermatology*, pp. 1755–85. (Oxford: Blackwell Scientific)
6. Degos, R. (1981). Maladie de Schaumann (sarcoïdose). In *Dermatologie,* (Paris: Flammarion Médecine-Sciences), pp. 529–40
7. Neville, E., Walker, A. N. and James, D. G. (1983). Prognostic factors predicting the outcome of sarcoidosis: an analysis of 818 patients. *Q. J. Med., new series LII,* **208,** 525–33
8. Besnier, E. (1889). Lupus pernio de la face; synovites fongueuses (scrofulo-

tuberculeuses symmétriques des extremites supérieures). *Annales de Dermatol. et de Syphiligraphie (Paris)*, **10,** 333–6
9. Willan, R. (1808). *On Cutaneous Diseases*. Vol. I. (London: J. Johnson)
10. Brewerton, D. A., Cockburn, C., James, D. G., and Neville, E. (1977). HLA antigens in sarcoidosis. *Clin. Exp. Immunol.*, **27,** 227–9
11. Caruthers, B., Day, T. B., Minus, H. R. and Young, R. C. (1975). Sarcoidosis: a comparison of cutaneous manifestations with chest radiographic changes. *J. Nat. Med. Assoc.*, **67,** 364–7
12. Black, M. M. (1985). Panniculitis. *J. Cut. Pathol.*, **12,** 366–80
13. Löfgren, S. (1946). Erythema nodosum: studies on etiology and pathogenesis in 185 adult cases. *Acta Med. Scand.*, Suppl. 174
14. Ridgway, H. A. and Ryan, T. J. (1981). Is micropapular sarcoidosis tuberculosis? *J. R. Soc. Med.*, **74,** 140–4
15. Rowland Payne, C. M. E., Meyrick Thomas, R. H. and Black, M. M. (1982). Sarcoïdes de Darier-Roussy ulcéreuses. *Journées Dermatologiques de Paris* cc 18
16. Mann, R. J. and Peachey, R. D. G. (1983). Sarcoidal tissue reaction—another complication of ear piercing. *Clin. Exp. Dermatol.*, **8,** 199–200
17. Rowland Payne, C. M. E., Meyrick Thomas, R. H. and Black, M. M. (1983). From silica granuloma to scar sarcoidosis. *Clin. Exp. Dermatol.*, **8,** 171–5
18. Spitieri, M. A., Matthey, F., Gordon, T., Carstairs, L. S. and James, D. G. (1985). Lupus pernio: a clinico-radiological study of 35 cases. *Br. J. Dermatol.*, **112,** 315–22
19. James, D. G., Neville, E. and Walker, A. (1975). Immunology of sarcoidosis. *Am. J. Med.*, **59,** 388–94
20. Sharma, O. P. and Balchum, O. J. (1972). Alcohol-induced pain and itching on hot showering in sarcoidosis: an unusual association. *Am. Rev. Resp. Dis.*, **106,** 763–6
21. Fong, Y. W. and Sharma, O. P. (1975). Pruritic maculopapular skin lesions in sarcoidosis. An unusual clinical presentation. *Arch. Dermatol.*, **111,** 362–4
22. Fagan, E. A., Moore-Gillon, J. C. and Turner-Warwick, M. (1983). Multiorgan granulomas and mitochondrial antibodies. *N. Engl. J. Med.*, **308,** 572–5
23. Degos, R., Lortat-Jacob, E., Delzant, O., Hewitt, J. and Labet, R. (1953). Maladie de Schaumann: Forme érythro-parakératosique (erythème sarcoïdique). Association à un prurigo nodularie (prurigo de la maladie de Schaumann?). *Bull de la Soc. de Dermatol. et de Syphiligraphie*, **60,** 410–12
24. Shmunes, E., Lantis, L. R. and Hurley, H. J. (1970). Verrucose sarcoidosis. *Arch. Dermatol.*, **102,** 665–9
25. Enjolras, O., Delrieu, F., Lessana-Lebowitch, M. and Escande, J. P. (1985). Une forme rare de sarcoïdose avec manifestations cutanées. *Journées Dermatologiques de Paris*, 1985, 169
26. Khan, F., Weasely, Z., Chasin, S. R. and Seriff, N. S. (1977). Conjunctival biopsy in sarcoidosis: a simple, safe and specific diagnostic procedure. *Ann. Ophthalmol.*, **9,** 671–6
27. Black, J. I. M. (1973). Sarcoidosis of the nose. *J. R. Soc. Med.*, **66,** 669–75
28. Baker, H. (1965). Atrophic alopecia due to granulomatous infiltration of the scalp in systemic sarcoidosis. *Proc. R. Soc. Med.*, **58,** 243–4
29. Bleehen, S. S. (1969). Systemic sarcoidosis with scalp involvement. *Proc. R. Soc. Med.*, **62,** 348–9

30. Felix, R. H. (1983). Alopecia of the shin – a presenting sign of sarcoidosis. *Br. J. Dermatol.*, **109** (Suppl. 24), 66
31. Greer, K. E., Harman, L. E. and Karne, A. L. (1977). Unusual cutaneous manifestations of sarcoidosis. *South. Med. J.*, **70**, 666–8
32. Appleyard, W. D. (1970). Sarcoidosis in a young child. *Proc. R. Soc. Med.*, **69**, 345
33. Carswell, W. A. (1972). A case of sarcoidosis presenting with erythema multiforme. *Am. Rev. Resp. Dis.*, **106**, 462–4
34. Beacham, B. E., Schuldenfrei, J. and Julka, S. S. (1984). Sarcoidosis presenting with erythema multiforme-like cutaneous lesions. *Cutis*, **33**, 461–3
35. Branford, W. A., Farr, P. M. and Porter, D. I. (1982). Annular vasculitis of the head and neck in a patient with sarcoidosis. *Br. J. Dermatol.*, **106**, 713–16
36. Rowland Payne, C. M. E. and McGibbon, D. H. (1985). Sarcoidosis presenting with widespread thrombophlebitis. *Clin. Exp. Dermatol.*, **10**, 592–4
37. Griffiths, C. E. M., Leonard, J. N. and Walker, M. M. (1986). Acquired ichthyosis and sarcoidosis. *Clin. Exp. Dermatol.*, **11**, 296–8
38. Clayton, R., Breathnach, A., Martin, B. and Feiwel, M. (1977). Hypopigmented sarcoidosis in the negro. Report of eight cases with ultrastructural observations. *Br. J. Dermatol.*, **96**, 119–25
39. Meyrick Thomas, R. H., McKee, P. H. and Black, M. M. (1981). Hypopigmented sarcoidosis. *J. R. Soc. Med.*, **74**, 921–3
40. Minus, H. R. and Grimes, P. E. (1983). Cutaneous manifestations of sarcoidosis in blacks. *Cutis*, **32**, 361–72
41. Bazex, A., Dupre, A., Christol, B., Cantala, P. and Bazex, J. (1970). Sarcoidosis with atrophic lesions and ulcers and the presence in some sarcoid granulomata of orceinophil fibres. *Br. J. Dermatol.*, **83**, 255–62
42. Neill, S. M., Smith, N. P. and Eady, R. A. J. (1984). Ulcerative sarcoidosis: a rare manifestation of a common disease. *Clin. Exp. Dermatol.*, **9**, 277–9
43. Morrison, J. G. L. (1974). Sarcoidosis in the Bantu: necrotizing and mutilating forms of the disease. *Br. J. Dermatol.*, **90**, 649–55
44. Muhlemann, M. F., Walker, N. P., Tan, L. B. and Champion, R. H. (1985). Elephantine sarcoidosis presenting as ulcerating lymphoedema. *J. R. Soc. Med.*, **78**, 260–1
45. Mann, R. J. and Allen, B. R. (1981). Nail dystrophy due to sarcoidosis. *Br. J. Dermatol.*, **105**, 599–601
46. Samman, P. D. and Fenton, D. A. (1986). *The Nails in Disease*, 4th Edn., pp. 85–86. (London: Heinemann Medical)
47. Tatnall, F. M., Barnes, H. M. and Sarkany, I. (1985). Sarcoidosis of the vulva. *Clin. Exp. Dermatol.*, **10**, 384–5
48. Goujon, C., Franc, M. P., Mauduit, G., Dorveaux, O. and Moulin, G. (1984). Maladie de Besnier-Boeck-Schaumann. Sarcoïdes multiples sur les régions exposées à la lumière. *Ann. Dermatol. Vénéréol.*, **111**, 815–17
49. Schnitzler, L. (1985). Maladie de Besnier-Boeck-Schaumann. Sarcöides saisonnières actiniques du visage: recul évolutif de 18 ans. *Ann. Dermatol. Vénéréol.*, **112**, 831–4
50. Wilson Jones, E. (1971). Necrobiosis lipoidica presenting on the face and scalp. *Trans. St John's Hosp. Dermatol. Soc.*, **57**, 202–20
51. Dahl, M. V. (1986). Is actinic granuloma really granuloma annulare? *Arch. Dermatol.*, **122**, 39–40

52. Muller, S. A. and Winkelmann, R. K. (1966). Necrobiosis lipoidica diabeticorum. *Arch. Dermatol.*, **94**, 1–10
53. Muhlemann, M. F. and Williams, D. R. R. (1984). Localised granuloma annulare is associated with insulin-dependent diabetes mellitus. *Br. J. Dermatol.*, **111**, 325–9
54. Umbert, P. and Winkelmann, R. K. (1977). Granuloma annulare and sarcoidosis. *Br. J. Dermatol.*, **97**, 481–6
55. Graham-Brown, R. A. C., Shuttleworth, D. and Sarkany, I. (1985). Coexistence of sarcoidosis and necrobiosis lipoidica of the legs – a report of 2 cases. *Clin. Exp. Dermatol.*, **10**, 274–8
56. Monk, B. E., and du Vivier, A. W. P. (1987). Necrobiosis lipoidica and sarcoidosis. *Clin. Exp. Dermatol.*, **12**, 294–5
57. Savin, J. (1969). Diabetes mellitus, sarcoidosis, ? necrobiosis lipoidica. *Proc. Soc. Med.*, **62**, 350
58. Saxe, N., Benetar, S. R., Bok, L. and Gordon, W. (1984). Sarcoidosis with leg ulcers and annular facial lesions. *Arch. Dermatol.*, **120**, 93–6
59. Fallahi, S., Deaver-Collins, R., Miller, R. K. and Halle, J. T. (1984). Coexistence of rheumatoid arthritis and sarcoidosis. *J. Rheumatol.*, **11**, 526–9
60. Burton, J. L. (1977). Granuloma annulare, rheumatoid nodules, and necrobiosis lipoidica. *Br. J. Dermatol.*, **97** (Suppl. 15), 52–4
61. Hanno, R., Needelman, A., Eiferman, R. A. and Callen, J. P. (1981). Cutaneous sarcoidal granulomas and the development of systemic sarcoidosis. *Arch. Dermatol.*, **117**, 203–7
62. Fulton, R. A. (1984). Psoriasiform sarcoidosis. *Br. J. Dermatol.*, **111** (Suppl. 26), 52–3
63. Wiesenhutter, C. W. and Sharma, D. P. (1979). Is sarcoidosis an autoimmune disease? A report of 4 cases and a review of the literature. *Semin. Arthritis Rheumatism*, **9**, 124–44
64. Seinfeld, E. D. and Sharma, O. P. (1983). TASS syndrome: unusual association of thyroiditis, Addison's disease, Sjögren's syndrome and sarcoidosis. *J. R. Soc. Med.*, **76**, 883–5
65. Thomas, L. L., Amberts, E. and Pegels, J. G. *et al.* (1982). Sarcoidosis associated with autoimmune thrombopenia and selective IgA deficiency. *Scand J. Haematol.*, **28**, 357–9
66. Sharvill, D. (1982). Lichen sclerosus, vitiligo, sarcoid reaction and macrocytic anaemia. Case presented to the Royal Society of Medicine, Section of Dermatology, 20th May 1982.

4

PORPHYRIA AND THE SKIN

G. H. ELDER

INTRODUCTION

The association between skin disease and excessive excretion of porphyrin has been known for over a century. In 1874, Baumstark showed that the urine of a patient with a bullous disorder, called pemphigus leprosus by Schultz, contained a red pigment that was similar to the haematoporphyrin that could be obtained by extracting blood with mineral acid. Subsequently, Gunther (1911) recognized that there was more than one type of cutaneous porphyria, while Meyer-Betz (1913), by injecting himself with haematoporphyrin, directly demonstrated that porphyrins are potent photosensitizing agents in man.

Over the last 70 years, increasingly sophisticated clinical and biochemical investigations have shown that the porphyrias are a group of disorders of haem biosynthesis in which characteristic clinical features occur in association with specific patterns of overproduction of porphyrins or their precursors. Each pattern of overproduction results from partial deficiency of one of the enzymes of the biosynthetic pathway (Fig. 4.1). The clinical features are of two types: acute attacks of porphyria, often precipitated by drugs and usually consisting of severe abdominal pain accompanied by neurological and psychiatric abnormalities; and skin lesions caused by porphyrin-induced photosensitization. Other disorders, such as lead poisoning, chronic alcoholism, and iron deficiency and other anaemias, in which abnormalities of porphyrin metabolism occur[1], are not associated with

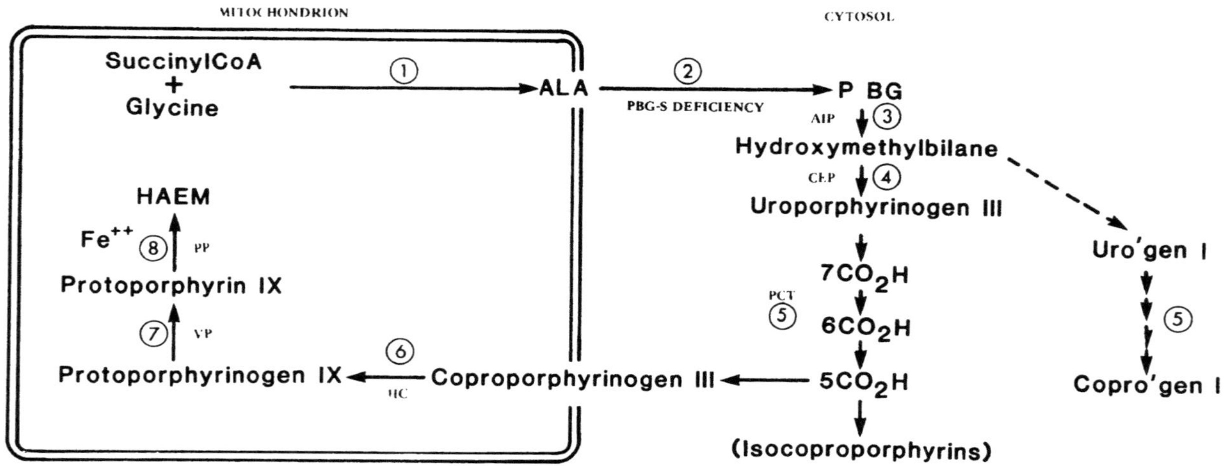

FIGURE 4.1 The pathway of haem biosynthesis. 1, 5-aminolaevulinate (ALA) synthase; 2, porphobilinogen (PBG) synthase; 3, PBG-deaminase; 4, uroporphyrinogen III synthase; 5, uroporphyrinogen decarboxylase; 6, coproporphyrinogen oxidase; 7, protoporphyrinogen oxidase; 8, ferrochelatase; 7–5CO_2H, hepta-, hexa- and pentacarboxylic porphyrinogens. Isocoproporphyrins are formed when pentacarboxylic porphyrinogen III accumulates in the cytosol. The non-enzymatic (– – –) conversion of hydroxymethylbilane to uroporphyrinogen I normally accounts for less than 1% of ALA utilization. Other abbreviations are as in Table 1

photosensitization and lack the distinctive clinical features of the porphyrias.

From the point of view of the clinical dermatologist, photosensitization induced by porphyrins needs to be distinguished from other photodermatoses and the type of porphyria identified; both these processes depend on selection and correct interpretation of the appropriate laboratory investigations. Identification of the type of porphyria is required for proper treatment and management of patients, and, since most of the porphyrias are inherited, for rational counselling of their relatives.

CLASSIFICATION

The main types of porphyria are listed in Table 4.1. In 1954, Schmid, Schwartz and Watson subdivided the porphyrias into hepatic and erythropoietic groups, according to whether haem precursors accumulated in the liver or the bone marrow. Although this subdivision is no longer considered to be absolute, it is still useful in practice to distinguish the hepatic porphyrias from the two other main types by measuring the concentration of free porphyrins in circulating erythrocytes (Table 4.1). Further subdivision into individual types depends largely on measurement of porphyrins and porphyrin precursors in urine, faeces and erythrocytes, since many of the diseases share the same clinical manifestations (Table 4.1).

The skin is unaffected in only two of the seven disorders listed in Table 4.1: acute intermittent porphyria and the very rare disease, porphobilinogen synthase deficiency. Because these conditions do not present to dermatologists, they will not be described here. Both have recently been reviewed[2,3].

PREVALENCE

All the porphyrias are uncommon conditions and few studies of their prevalence have been carried out. Some estimates are given in Table

TABLE 4.1 The main types of porphyria

Disorder	*Clinical features*		*Estimated prevalence of overt porphyria*
	Acute attacks	*Photosensitization*	
A. Porphyrias with increased erythrocyte porphyrin concentrations			
Congenital erythropoietic porphyria (CEP)	–	+	<1 : 10^6
Protoporphyria (PP)	–	+	1 : 200 000
B. Hepatic porphyrias; erythrocyte porphyrin concentration normal			
Porphyria cutanea tarda (PCT)	–	+	1 : 25 000
Acute hepatic porphyrias			
Acute intermittent porphyria (AIP)	+	–	1–2 : 100 000
Hereditary coproporphyria (HC)	+	+	
Variegate porphyria (VP)	+	+	1 : 250 000
PBG-synthase deficiency	+	–	

4.1, where the figures refer to patients with overt porphyria; latent and subclinical porphyria is commoner. The prevalence of the most frequent porphyria, porphyria cutanea tarda (PCT), varies from country to country. It seems to be most frequent in Spain, Italy and central and eastern Europe, the prevalence in Czechoslovakia being 1 : 7000. In the autosomal dominant acute hepatic porphyrias, founder effects also lead to geographical differences: in South Africa, an estimated 30 000 carriers of the gene for variegate porphyria descend from one immigrant who reached the Cape in the late seventeenth century.

METABOLIC ABNORMALITIES

Each of the seven porphyrias listed in Table 4.1 results from partial deficiency of a different enzyme of the pathway of haem biosynthesis

(Fig. 4.1). The rate of haem biosynthesis is controlled by the activity of 5-amino-laevulinate (ALA) synthase, the enzyme that catalyses the formation of the first intermediate of the pathway. The activity of ALA-synthase is largely determined by the concentration of haem in a regulatory haem pool; a decrease in concentration leads to an increase in activity and vice versa. Under normal conditions, the concentrations of the substrates of the enzymes that convert ALA to haem are well below those required for maximum activity of the respective enzymes. Partial deficiency of one of these enzymes decreases the rate of haem synthesis, depletes the regulatory haem pool and thereby increases the activity of ALA-synthase. The increase in ALA-synthase activity leads to an increase in the concentration of the substrate of the defective enzyme until a new steady state is reached at which the rate of haem synthesis is restored to normal. Thus the porphyrias, although disorders of haem biosynthesis, are not associated with defective haem formation, except in the liver during attacks of acute porphyria, when the compensatory mechanism outlined above temporarily fails.

When the substrate of the defective enzyme is either a porphyrin, a porphyrinogen that rapidly autoxidizes to a porphyrin within the tissues, or hydroxymethylbilane that undergoes non-enzymatic cyclization to a porphyrin, porphyrins may be produced in sufficient excess to induce photosensitization. Thus the skin is affected only in those porphyrias in which enzymes distal to the formation of hydroxymethylbilane are affected (Fig. 4.1). In a sense, skin lesions are the price that is paid for maintaining normal rates of haem formation. The patterns of overproduction of porphyrins and porphyrin precursors in the porphyrias are shown in Table 4.2.

Haem biosynthesis occurs in all nucleated cells. In humans, about 75% of the haem synthesized each day is produced in the bone marrow; most of the rest being made in the liver, largely for the synthesis of the cytochrome P-450 component of the microsomal mixed-function oxygenase system that is responsible for the metabolism of a wide variety of drugs, foreign chemicals and endogenous compounds. With the exception of some types of PCT, the enzyme defects in the cutaneous porphyrias are present in all tissues. However the compensatory changes outlined above do not occur in all tissues. For example, the enzyme defects that underlie the hepatic porphyrias

TABLE 4.2 Overproduction of haem precursors in clinically overt porphyria

Disorder	*Increased excretion of:*	*Increased erythrocyte concentration of:*
PBG-synthase deficiency	ALA; coproporphyrin III (urine only)	Zinc-protoporphyrin
AIP	PBG>ALA (urine only)	—
CEP	Uroporphyrin I, coproporphyrin I	Uro-, copro-, zinc-protoporphyrin
PCT	Uroporphyrin I and III, hepta-, hexa- and pentacarboxylic porphyrins, isocoproporphyrins	—
HC	PBG*>ALA; coproporphyrin III	—
VP	PBG*>ALA; protoporphyrin IX>coproporphyrin III; X-porphyrin	—
PP	± protoporphyrin IX	Free protoporphyrin

* In HC and VP urinary PBG, ALA may be normal except during an acute attack of porphyria. X-porphyrin is a hydrophilic porphyrin (probably a group of dicarboxylic porphyrin–peptide conjugates) excreted in the bile in VP.

(Table 4.1) increase ALA-synthase activity and substrate production only in the liver; the reason for this is not fully understood. There is also considerable variation between individuals in the way in which they respond to quantitatively similar enzyme defects. Some may have no detectable increase in substrate concentration, while others have severe clinical porphyria. Part of this variation is determined by interaction between the enzyme defect and external, acquired factors. Thus, in the acute hepatic porphyrias, acute attacks of porphyria may be provoked by barbiturates and other drugs that induce cytochrome P-450 synthesis in the liver by stimulating the demand for haem for assembly of additional cytochrome molecules. However, even in the acute hepatic porphyrias, there are many aspects of the relationship between the enzyme defect and substrate overproduction that remain obscure.

BIOCHEMICAL GENETICS

Apart from some types of PCT, all the main types of human porphyrias show clearly defined patterns of inheritance (Table 4.3); there is no evidence that any cases are the result of new mutations. In all but one of the autosomal dominant porphyrias the activity of the defective enzyme is decreased by 40–50% in all tissues, a finding that is compatible with inheritance of one normal allele that produces its normal quota of active enzyme, and one mutant allele that is either silent or encodes an unstable or largely inactive enzyme protein. The one exception is protoporphyria (erythropoietic protoporphyria), in which the activity of ferrochelatase is decreased by at least 75%, indicating that the mutation may interfere in some way with expression of the normal allele.

In recent years a number of cutaneous porphyrias have been identified in which at least some patients appear to be homozygous for the mutant genes that, in a single dose, produce the autosomal dominant cutaneous porphyrias (Table 4.4). In these homozygous forms, enzyme activities are usually less than 20% of normal and the clinical features tend to be more severe and to develop earlier than in their autosomal dominant counterparts. Study of these very rare diseases, particularly hepatoerythropoietic porphyria[4], which, with homozygous variegate porphyria[5], is probably the most frequent type, suggests that each of the inherited cutaneous porphyrias is likely to be genetically het-

TABLE 4.3 Inherited porphyrias

Disorder	*Chromosomal location of defective gene*	*Mode of inheritance*
PBG synthase deficiency	9	Autosomal recessive
AIP	11q24-ter	Autosomal dominant
CEP	Unknown	Autosomal recessive
PCT (type II familial)	1p34	Autosomal dominant
HC	9	Autosomal dominant
VP	Unknown	Autosomal dominant
PP	Unknown	Autosomal dominant

TABLE 4.4 Homozygous forms of autosomal dominant porphyrias

Disorder	*Enzyme deficiency*	*Per cent control activity*	*Autosomal dominant counterpart*
Hepatoerythropoietic porphyria	Uroporphyrinogen decarboxylase	3–24	PCT (type II)
Homozygous hereditary coproporphyria	Coproporphyrinogen oxidase	2	HC
Harderoporphyria	Coproporphyrinogen oxidase	10	HC
Homozygous variegate porphyria	Protoporphyrinogen oxidase	5–14	VP
Homozygous protoporphyria	Ferrochelatase	less than 10	PP

erogeneous, with different mutations giving rise to the same phenotype, as has already been demonstrated for acute intermittent porphyria[6].

As might be predicted, the two types of porphyria that show an autosomal recessive pattern of inheritance are both very uncommon disorders. In CEP, the activity of uroporphyrinogen III synthase is decreased by 80% or more and there is even less residual activity in PBG-synthase deficiency. In PBG-synthase deficiency a structurally abnormal enzyme with low catalytic activity is produced, but the molecular basis of the low enzyme activity in CEP has not yet been defined.

PHOTOSENSITIZATION BY PORPHYRINS

Clinical features

Two types of skin reaction are seen in the cutaneous porphyrias: acute photosensitivity, and a group of changes that include increased mechanical fragility of the skin and subepidermal blisters as the commonest manifestations. Both are restricted to areas of the skin that are exposed to sunlight. The first is the main feature of protoporphyria, while the second characterizes PCT and all other cutaneous porphyrias. These two types of reaction are so distinct that there is rarely any clinical confusion between protoporphyria and other kinds of porphyria. However, they both reflect porphyrin-induced photo-damage to the skin, their underlying pathology is similar, and there is no absolute distinction between them. For example, acute photosensitivity in PCT and blisters in protoporphyria are both rare but well recognized.

In protoporphyria, an intense pricking, itching and burning sensation develops, usually within 5–30 minutes after exposure to sunlight although it is occasionally delayed for as long as 4 hours. The initial sensations blend into severe, burning pain in sun-exposed areas. The severity of visible skin changes varies. Erythema is often accompanied by oedema. Crusting and petechiae may develop later. Less common acute lesions include photo-onycholysis, with eventual shedding of the nails, and small vesicles; larger bullae and skin fragility are rare. The

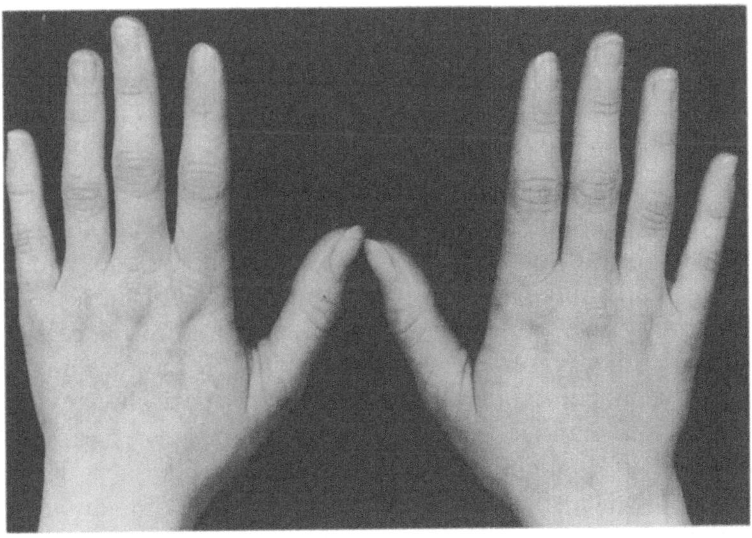

FIGURE 4.2 Erythropoietic protoporphyria. Waxy thickening of the skin over the metacarpophalangeal joints can be seen

skin may appear normal between attacks, but with repeated episodes some chronic changes usually develop: the skin becomes thickened, pitted with small linear or circular scars, and may appear waxy (Fig. 4.2). The face, especially the bridge of the nose, and the backs of the hands over the metacarpophalangeal and interphalangeal joints are common sites for these changes.

In the other cutaneous porphyrias, exemplified by PCT, acute photosensitivity is rare, the lesions usually produce no more than inconvenience or discomfort, and the patient often fails to notice any relationship between their appearance and exposure to sunlight. Four features are common: skin fragility, bullae, hypertrichosis and pigmentation (Fig. 4.3). Increased fragility is almost always present and is usually the first abnormality to appear. Minor trauma dislodges small areas of epidermis to produce erosions, seen most frequently on those areas of sun-exposed skin, such as the knuckles, that receive the most trauma. The erosions heal slowly with crusting, scarring and milia formation. Secondary infection often delays healing. Subepidermal bullae either appear spontaneously or after minor mechanical or heat injury. They usually contain clear fluid but may be haemorrhagic. They eventually rupture and heal in the same way as erosions.

The long-term effects of these changes are very variable. A brief episode of PCT may leave no more than a few residual scars that are only apparent on close examination. In contrast, repeated erosions, bullae and secondary infection over several years may produce severe photomutilation with extensive scarring of sun-exposed skin, resorption of the terminal phalanges, loss of nasal and aural cartilage, severe scarring and contraction of the eyelids and lips and pigmented, dystrophic nails, which may be lost through photo-onycholysis.

Hypertrichosis is present in many patients and may occasionally be the presenting feature. Excess hair grows on the face and arms, particularly extending laterally from the eyebrows. The new growth consists of long, lanugo-type, dark hair and may be excessive, as in the outbreak of hexachlorobenzene-induced porphyria in Turkey in the late 1950s when affected children were known as 'monkey' children. Pigmentation is the least frequent of the four common skin changes. It may be diffuse or patchy and is most prominent on the face and hands. Occasionally areas of hypopigmentation develop in scarred areas of skin.

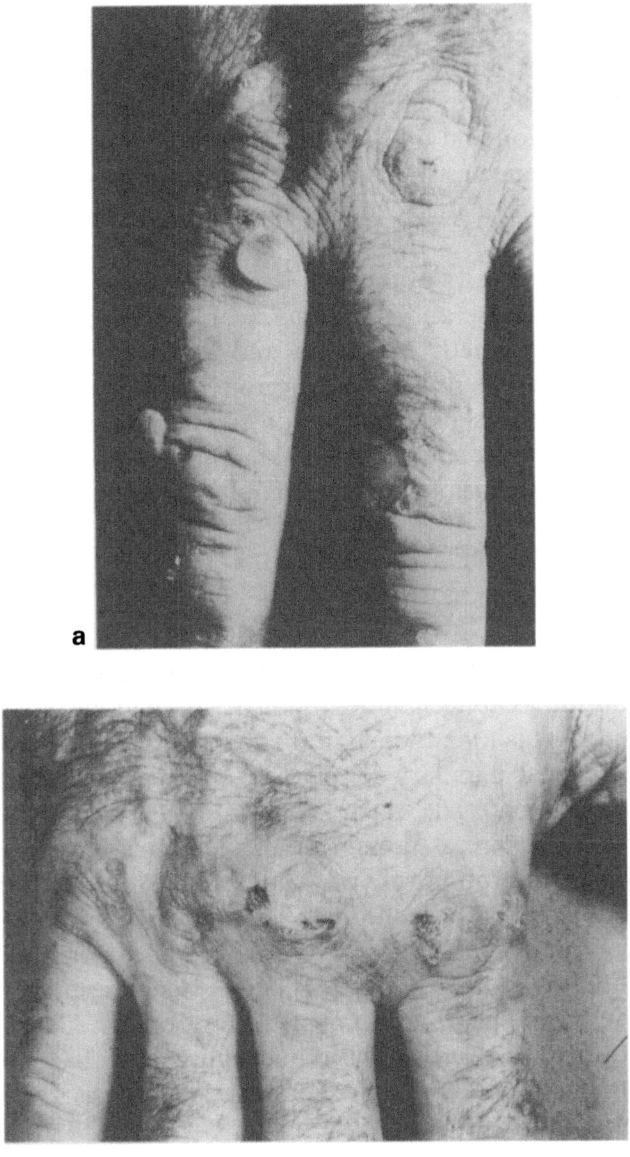

a

b

FIGURE 4.3 Porphyria cutanea tarda. (**a**) An intact bulla is visible; (**b**) Erosions can be seen

Other skin manifestations are less common. Scleroderma-like lesions may occur on the face, neck, scalp and thorax, even in the absence of exposure to sunlight, and become calcified, especially in the pre-auricular region and on the scalp. Scarring alopecia, centrofacial papular lymphangiectasis and various ocular lesions, including penetrating ulceration of the sclera, have also been described in severe cutaneous porphyria.

In general the severity of the skin lesions depends on the nature of the underlying disease and the amount of exposure to sunlight. In congenital erythropoietic porphyria and hepatoerythropoietic porphyria, where there is persistent overproduction of porphyrins from an early age, severe skin damage with photomutilation is usual. In PCT, the more severe and unusual skin changes are seen more frequently in Mediterranean countries than in northern Europe.

Histopathology

In all cutaneous porphyrias, histological examination of sun-exposed areas of skin shows abnormalities in the dermis and lower epidermis[7]. Homogeneous, eosinophilic material is deposited in and around the blood vessels in the papillary dermis and, in severe cases, elsewhere in the dermis. This material, which stains with PAS and is resistant to digestion with diastase, is present in all cutaneous porphyrias but is most prominent in protoporphyria. The same hyaline deposits thicken the basement membrane zone between the dermis and epidermis. Bullae occur sub-epidermally above this thickened zone and dermal papillae, stiffened by hyaline deposits, may extend irregularly into the cavity, giving an appearance known as 'festooning'. Other changes that occur include sclerosis with thickening of collagen bundles, especially in old lesions, and hyperkeratosis, acanthosis and increased numbers of granular cells in the dermis.

Direct immunofluorescence reveals the presence of IgG and other plasma components around the walls of the blood vessels and at the epidermo-dermal junction, indicating leakage of intravascular proteins from damaged capillaries.

Mechanisms

Three factors are required for the production of skin damage in the porphyrias: accumulation of porphyrins in cutaneous tissues, light and oxygen[8,9].

Monochromator experiments show an action spectrum for erythema in patients with cutaneous porphyrias that closely resembles the electronic absorption spectrum of neutral porphyrins; the greatest damage is produced by wavelengths in the 400–410 nm region corresponding to the main or Soret absorption peak. Light of this wavelength is not shielded by window glass as is the ultraviolet radiation that causes sunburn and other photo-effects in normal individuals and in those sensitized by compounds other than porphyrins.

The way in which light interacts with porphyrins to cause tissue damage has been the subject of much research[8–10]. The initial reaction appears to be a porphyrin-catalysed activation of molecular oxygen to form chemically reactive species. Absorption of light produces singlet excited-state porphyrins that either decay to the ground state with emission of red light (fluorescence) or convert to relatively long-lived triplet states. Triplet porphyrins react with molecular oxygen to give singlet excited oxygen and, much less efficiently, some superoxide radical anion. Both singlet oxygen and the hydroxyl radicals that may be generated in subsequent reactions are chemically highly reactive. Evidence that singlet oxygen has a major role in the photodynamic action of porphyrins comes from the observation that high concentrations of β-carotene, which quench the production of singlet oxygen, are effective in the prevention of acute photosensitivity in the porphyrias.

The main targets in the skin for these reactive oxygen species have not been identified. Lipid-containing cell membranes appear to be particularly susceptible to photo-damage, but proteins and nucleic acids can also become modified. Release of lysosomal contents is probably a secondary event rather than a primary initiator of the changes in the skin. *In vitro* experiments have shown that porphyrins can catalyse the photoactivation of complement and this effect may contribute to the inflammatory response. Since singlet oxygen and hydroxyl radicals have lifetimes of only a few microseconds, they produce damage close to the site at which they are generated. The porphyrins that accumulate in the different porphyrias differ in their solubility properties and thus are localized at different sites within cells. For example, protoporphyrin, which is lipophilic, tends to associate with lipid-containing membranes. This difference in distribution, and hence in the site of production of toxic oxygen metabolites, may help to explain the striking clinical difference between protoporphyria, in which protoporphyrin accumulates, and the other cutaneous porphyrias, in which the major circulating porphyrins are more hydrophilic.

Porphyrins may also produce pathological changes in the absence of light. Thus uroporphyrin stimulates the production of collagen by fibroblasts in the dark; this response may be related to the sclerodermatous changes in PCT. More importantly, evidence is accumulating that prolonged exposure of hepatocytes to excess porphyrins leads to an increased incidence of hepatocellular carcinoma[11].

CLINICAL FEATURES OF THE CUTANEOUS PORPHYRIAS

Congenital erythropoietic porphyria (Gunther's disease)

This uncommon porphyria results from partial deficiency of uroporphyrinogen III synthase (Fig. 4.1), which leads to the overproduction, particularly in erythroid cells, of large amounts of isomer series I porphyrins derived from the non-enzymatic cyclization of hydroxymethylbilane to uroporphyrinogen III. There are two forms: the classical type that starts in infancy and a late-onset variant[12].

Gunther's disease typically presents in infancy when either red urine, due to excessive excretion of porphyrins, or photosensitivity with the subsequent appearance of bullae is noticed. This is the type of bullous porphyria in which the skin lesions described above are seen at their most severe; extensive scarring and photomutilation is usual in older patients. A characteristic clinical sign is a brown discoloration of the teeth, or erythrodontia, due to deposition of porphyrin in bone. The teeth show a bright red fluorescence when examined with a Wood's lamp.

Some degree of anaemia is present in many patients. Fluorescence microscopy of the bone marrow shows red fluorescence in a proportion of normoblasts and these develop into erythrocytes that contain increased concentrations of uroporphyrin and other porphyrins. This abnormality is associated with a shortened life span, probably because the porphyrin catalyses photo-damage of the red cell membrane in superficial capillaries. The ensuing haemolytic anaemia is usually mild and well-compensated, but it may be severe and even life-threatening; the clinical course is often intermittent. Splenomegaly is a frequent finding.

The late-onset form of the disease is much less severe. The few patients who have been encountered since it was first recognized in 1965 have all been clinically indistinguishable from PCT cases, apart from splenomegaly with mild haemolytic anaemia in some. All have been adults, ranging in age from the third to the sixth decades. Recent experience in the author's department suggests that this condition, because of its similarity to PCT, is underdiagnosed and may be more frequent than has been appreciated.

Porphyria cutanea tarda (PCT)

Definition and pathogenesis

PCT is a syndrome in which skin lesions (Fig. 4.3) indistinguishable from those of other cutaneous porphyrias, apart from protoporphyria, occur in association with a characteristic pattern of porphyrin overproduction that results from decreased activity of uroporphyrinogen decarboxylase in the liver (Fig. 4.1). In contrast to other types of porphyria, there is more than one cause of the enzyme defect. About 70–80% of patients have type I or sporadic PCT in which there is no family history of porphyria and no evidence of exposure to porphyrogenic chemicals and in which the enzyme defect is restricted to the liver. The cause of the hepatic enzyme defect in type I PCT is unknown. There is some evidence that the process that produces it is reversible and may be iron-dependent[13], but the role of the liver cell damage, particularly due to alcohol, that is so frequently associated with PCT has not been established. Most of the remaining patients have type II or familial PCT, in which the enzyme defect is inherited as an autosomal dominant trait that is expressed in all tissues; only a minority of gene carriers have overt PCT, so a family history of PCT is often absent. Finally, PCT may be produced by exposure to a toxic chemical that predictably decreases hepatic uroporphyrinogen decarboxylase activity. The best known of these is hexachlorobenzene, which was responsible for porphyria turcica[14] but 2,3,7,8-tetrachlorodibenzo-*p*-dioxin has also been reported to cause human porphyria.

Clinical features

PCT is typically a disease of middle-aged men who drink too much alcohol, but in recent years this picture has changed with a fall in the age of onset and an increase in the frequency of PCT in women[15]. Although largely due to the importance of oestrogens, including those used for oral contraception, as aetiological agents[15], this change probably also reflects an altered pattern of alcohol consumption. Most patients present with blisters and a history of preceding mechanical fragility of the skin; occasionally hypertrichosis is the first sign or the condition may be recognized incidentally in patients with alcoholic liver disease or some other disorder associated with PCT. Alcohol or oestrogens can be identified as aetiological agents in about 80% of patients[15]. Less commonly, PCT may be associated with other types of liver disease, including viral hepatitis, or with systemic lupus erythematosus and may occasionally occur in patients undergoing chronic haemodialysis. About 15% of patients with PCT have non-insulin-dependent diabetes mellitus.

Clinical evidence of liver disease is uncommon, but minor abnormalities of liver function, especially increased plasma aspartate transaminase activities, are present in most patients. Needle biopsy of the liver usually shows some degree of liver cell damage, ranging from fatty infiltration and piecemeal necrosis with minor periportal inflammatory changes in the majority to frank cirrhosis in some, especially those with a long history of skin lesions[16]. Hepatocytes contain large amounts of uroporphyrin and heptacarboxylic porphyrin that can be seen either by light microscopy as needle-like crystals or as red fluorescence of the biopsy core in ultraviolet light.

Because of the effectiveness of venesection as a treatment (see below), iron metabolism has been extensively studied in PCT. In most series, around 90% of patients have had mild to moderate hepatic siderosis, although this figure may be biased by selection of the more severely affected patients for biopsy. Hepatic non-haem iron concentrations are increased in about 60% and total body iron stores in about two thirds of patients. However, it is clear that individuals with no detectable abnormality of iron metabolism can develop PCT. The available evidence indicates that PCT is an iron-dependent disease; it does not occur in iron-deficient subjects and requires at least normal hepatic iron stores to develop. The onset of PCT in susceptible individuals may be accelerated by iron-overload, but the rarity of PCT in haemochromatosis suggests that iron-overload does not directly cause PCT. At present there is no firm evidence that heterozygosity for haemochromatosis is an important cause of hepatic siderosis in PCT.

It is not usually possible to distinguish between type I and type II PCT except by measurement of erythrocyte uroporphyrinogen decarboxylase and appropriate family studies. Onset before the age of twenty strongly suggests type II PCT. After this age, about 20% of patients will have the type II disorder. A family history of PCT, especially in a young patient, is also indicative of the type II form, but its absence is of little diagnostic value as the majority of type II patients have no relatives with the disorder. In addition, a number of families have recently been identified that contain more than one individual with a form of PCT that is biochemically and clinically indistinguishable from the type I disorder, showing that familial PCT is heterogeneous.

The prognosis of PCT appears to depend on the nature and severity of the underlying liver disease. Long-term follow-up has shown an increased frequency of hepatocellular carcinoma in untreated patients[11].

Acute hepatic porphyrias

Each type of acute hepatic porphyria may present with an acute neuropsychiatric attack (Table 4.1). The clinical features of these attacks of acute porphyria, which may be precipitated by drugs, alcohol or fasting and which may end fatally, have been reviewed[2] and will not be discussed here.

Skin lesions occur in two types of acute hepatic porphria: variegate porphyria and hereditary coproporphyria (Table 4.1). In both conditions, skin lesions may be the only clinical manifestation or they may occur in conjunction with an attack of acute porphyria. The changes in the skin are indistinguishable from those seen in PCT. Neither condition occurs before puberty.

In the United Kingdom, variegate porphyria usually presents with skin lesions alone. It is then often clinically indistinguishable from PCT because only a minority of patients have a family history of acute porphyria. Less commonly, patients present with acute porphyria that is accompanied by skin changes, especially evidence of increased fragility, in about half the cases.

Hereditary coproporphyria is seen less frequently than the other acute hepatic porphyrias. Patients usually present with acute porphyria, minor skin changes being present in about one third of cases. In both hereditary coproporphyria and variegate porphyria, skin lesions without acute porphyria may be precipitated by an episode of intercurrent cholestasis, which reduces biliary excretion of porphyrin and thereby increases porphyrin concentrations in plasma and tissues.

Protoporphyria

Protoporphyria (erythropoietic protoporphyria, erythrohepatic protoporphyria) results from decreased activity of ferrochelatase, the enzyme that inserts iron into protoporphyrin to make haem. As a consequence, protoporphyrin accumulates in erythroid cells and in the liver. Protoporphyrin from both sources leaks into the plasma and thus reaches the skin.

Overproduction of protoporphyrin has three clinical consequences[17]. First, it causes acute photosensitivity of the type already described (Fig. 4.2). Patients usually present in early childhood and both sexes are affected equally. Older patients may be strikingly pale owing to assiduous avoidance of sunlight. Second, protoporphyrin may crystallize in the bile and lead to the formation of gallstones, which occur in about 15% of patients, usually during the third and fourth decades. Third, protoporphyrin may accumulate in the liver, where it is deposited as crystals. In the majority of patients this has no clinical consequences, but a minority develop abnormalities of liver function that may herald the onset of liver failure. This complication, although rare, may occur at any age and invariably progresses rapidly[18].

Although the condition is inherited as an autosomal dominant trait, clinical penetrance is low and many patients have no family history of the disease.

Accumulation of protoporphyrin in erythrocytes does not lead to haemolytic anaemia, as does uroporphyrin in congenital erythropoietic porphyria, but ferrochelatase deficiency does seem to impair erythroid haem synthesis so that many patients have a mild to moderate microcytic anaemia.

DIAGNOSIS OF THE CUTANEOUS PORPHYRIAS

In order to establish that skin lesions are caused by porphyria, it is necessary to show that they are associated with an appropriate pattern of overproduction of porphyrins. Conversely, exclusion of porphyria as the cause of skin lesions requires demonstration that there is no increased production of porphyrins. Selection and correct interpretation of laboratory investigations for these purposes depends on knowledge of the clinical features. In dermatological practice, porphyrias usually present in one of three ways: as acute photosensitivity without blisters or fragile skin, as a PCT-like syndrome in adults, or as a PCT-like syndrome in children.

Acute photosensitivity

The only type of porphyria that presents as acute photosensitivity without blisters or fragile skin is protoporphyria. This condition can be differentiated from all other causes of photosensitivity by demonstrating an increased concentration of protoporphyrin in erythrocytes. A normal erythrocyte protoporphyrin concentration excludes protoporphyria as the cause of photosensitivity. The most useful front-line test is measurement of total erythrocyte porphyrin by one of the rapid fluorometric micromethods that have been described[19]. If this test is not available, screening procedures using solvent extraction or fluorescence[20] may be used, but both tests give occasional false negatives so, when clinical suspicion is strong, negative screening tests need to be confirmed by quantitative methods.

An increased erythrocyte porphyrin concentration in a patient with photosensitivity does not by itself prove protoporphyria. Total erythrocyte porphyrin concentration is also increased in other conditions, notably iron deficiency, lead poisoning and some anaemias, although concentrations are usually lower than in many cases of protoporphyria. However, in these conditions, as in normal subjects, the erythrocyte porphyrin is almost entirely zinc-protoporphyrin, which remains within the red cells so that plasma porphyrin concentrations are normal. In protoporphyria, the erythrocyte porphyrin is almost entirely free protoporphyrin and the same compound is found in the plasma.

Urinary porphyrin excretion is normal in protoporphyria, except in some patients with terminal liver failure, but faecal excretion of protoporphyrin may be increased. Since faecal porphyrin excretion is normal in about 40% of patients, measurement of porphyrin excretion should never be used as the only test when searching for this condition.

PCT-type skin lesions in adults

The porphyrias that present as PCT-type skin lesions in adults are listed in Table 4.5 in approximate order of frequency. Very rarely this type of porphyria may be caused by a tumour, usually an adenoma, that arises in an otherwise normal liver and secretes large amounts of porphyrins. This possibility should always be considered in the differential diagnosis of PCT, particularly if the porphyrin excretion pattern is atypical.

The porphyrias in this group can be differentiated by measurement of porphyrin precursors and porphyrins in urine, and porphyrins in faeces (Table 4.5). All are associated with an increased urinary porphyrin concentration. In some patients, there may be sufficient porphyrins to colour the urine red, or to show red fluorescence when the urine is viewed in ultraviolet light from a Wood's lamp; in others the urine may look normal. Simple screening tests based on extraction

TABLE 4.5 PCT-type skin lesions in adults

	Laboratory differentiation				
			Main porphyrins in:		
Disorder	*Increased RBC porphyrin*	*Increased urine PBG*	*Urine*	*Faeces*	*Plasma porphyrin fluorescence (emission max.)*
PCT	–	–	URO> HEPTA	ISOCOPRO, HEPTA	615 nm
VP	–	±	Variable	PROTO> COPRO	626 nm
CEP	+	–	URO I, COPRO I	COPRO I	615 nm
HC	–	±	COPRO III	COPRO III	615 nm
Hepatoma	–	–	Variable	Variable	
Pseudoporphyria	–	–	Normal	Normal	*Not present

* Plasma uroporphyrin (615 nm) may be increased in patients with chronic renal failure and bullous dermatosis

of urinary porphyrins into organic solvents[19] are widely used to screen for these porphyrias. It is important to realize that these tests are insensitive and may occasionally fail to detect patients with porphyria, particularly those who are first seen in remission or when their skin lesions are beginning to heal. In order to establish a diagnosis, quantitative analysis of individual porphyrins in both urine and faeces is required (Table 4.5). Measurement of urinary porphyrins alone is not sufficient. The urine of some patients with variegate porphyria has a porphyrin composition that is identical to that of PCT; the late-onset form of congenital erythropoietic porphyria may also be difficult to distinguish from PCT by urine analysis.

Poh-Fitzpatrick has described a useful, rapid test for the diagnosis of cutaneous porphyrias[21]. In patients with active skin lesions, fluorescence spectroscopy of plasma diluted 1 : 10 with phosphate-buffered saline shows an emission peak due to porphyrins at a wavelength that is determined by the nature of the porphyrins. This test enables variegate porphyria to be differentiated from PCT and other cutaneous porphyrias (Table 4.5). Furthermore, if no porphyrin is detected, it strongly suggests that the skin lesions are not caused by porphyria.

Skin reactions to some drugs (nalidixic acid, naproxen), the bullous dermatosis seen in chronic haemodialysis, and some other conditions may be clinically indistinguishable from PCT[22]. These so-called 'pseudoporphyrias' can be differentiated from porphyria only by showing that porphyrin excretion and erythrocyte porphyrin concentrations are normal. For this purpose, quantitative measurement with estimation of individual porphyrins is essential. In patients undergoing long-term haemodialysis, PCT is best differentiated from non-porphyric bullous dermatosis by measuring isocoproporphyrin in faeces; plasma measurements are unreliable, as the concentration of uroporphyrin is increased in renal failure.

PCT-type skin lesions in children

Skin lesions of PCT type are rare in children. They may be caused by congenital erythropoietic porphyria, PCT, hepatoerythropoietic porphyria, homozygous variegate porphyria or homozygous forms of hereditary coproporphyria. Porphyrin excretion patterns are similar to those of the corresponding adult disorders (Table 4.2). In addition, erythrocyte porphyrin concentrations are increased in all these conditions, except PCT. Final diagnosis of hepatoerythropoietic porphyria and the homozygous counterparts of the acute hepatic porphyrias requires measurement of the activity of the defective enzymes.

Diagnosis of latent porphyria

Identification of asymptomatic relatives who have inherited porphyria is obligatory in variegate porphyria and hereditary coproporphyria

TABLE 4.6 Detection of latent cutaneous porphyrias

Disorder	*Laboratory investigations*
VP	Faecal PROTO, COPRO; plasma porphyrin; protoporphyrinogen oxidase (lymphocytes, fibroblasts)
HC	Faecal COPRO; coproporphyrinogen oxidase (lymphocytes, fibroblasts)
PCT	Urine URO, HEPTA; faecal ISOCOPRO, HEPTA; uroporphyrinogen decarboxylase (erythrocytes)
PP	Erythrocyte free PROTO; ferrochelatase (lymphocytes, fibroblasts)

(see below) and may be required in protoporphyria and PCT. The appropriate investigations are listed in Table 4.6. Enzyme measurements, which are complex and time-consuming, should be reserved for those individuals in whom porphyrin analyses give either normal or equivocal results.

MANAGEMENT OF THE CUTANEOUS PORPHYRIAS

The treatment of the porphyrias has been reviewed[23,24] and only selected aspects will be described here. PCT is the only form of cutaneous porphyria for which specific treatments that produce clinical remission and return the biochemical abnormalities associated with overt disease to normal have been introduced. In all others, treatment depends on prevention of light-induced skin damage by various strategies, which tend to be least effective in those conditions, such as congenital erythropoietic porphyria[12], where overproduction of porphyrins is most severe and sustained.

Prevention of light-induced skin damage

There are three approaches to prevention of light-induced skin damage in porphyria: physical avoidance of sunlight, the use of sunscreen ointments and the accumulation of a protective layer of β-carotene in the skin. The wavelengths (around 400 nm) that cause most damage are not blocked by most sunscreen preparations. Even reflectant or combined absorbent/reflectant preparations with high sun-protection factors (SPF about 10–15) are often ineffective and the quantities of these opaque creams that need to be applied may be cosmetically unacceptable. Oral administration of β-carotene is often effective in protoporphyria and may be useful in other cutaneous porphyrias. The usual dose is 60–180 mg/day and enough should be given to produce a serum carotene concentration of at least 600–800 μg/decilitre. At this concentration, the skin takes on a yellowish tinge but there are no significant side-effects. The β-carotene in the skin appears to prevent photo-damage by acting as a singlet-oxygen and free-radical trap; blood porphyrin concentrations are not altered.

Liver disease in protoporphyria

Although severe liver disease is uncommon in protoporphyria, it may appear in any patient at any age. At present, there is no reliable method for either its prediction or its prevention. Very high erythrocyte and plasma protoporphyrin concentrations and biochemical abnormalities of liver function may all indicate patients who are at risk, and who may require needle biopsy of the liver for assessment. In such patients, attempts to prevent or slow the development of liver disease are worthwhile, the objectives being to decrease protoporphyrin production and to lower the amount of porphyrin stored in the liver. Correction of any iron-deficiency that may be present is helpful. Manœuvres such as overtransfusion and the intravenous administration of haematin appear to decrease porphyrin formation but are not suitable for long-term treatment. An alternative approach is to attempt to interrupt the enterohepatic circulation of protoporphyrin with oral cholestyramine or activated charcoal preparations. Recently, chenodeoxycholic acid has been reported to decrease the excretion and hepatic production of protoporphyrin, but its therapeutic effectiveness has not yet been fully evaluated[24]. For those patients who develop acute hepatic failure, the only treatment appears to be liver transplantation.

Treatment of PCT

Withdrawal of alcohol or oestrogens may lead to clinical remission in those patients in whom these aetiological agents are implicated. However, remission is often slow to follow withdrawal and may not occur. So, particularly when skin lesions are troublesome, it is frequently preferable to use one of the two specific treatments, venesection or chloroquine, that are almost always successful in PCT but always ineffective in the other cutaneous porphyrias.

Venesection therapy induces prolonged remission with reversal of biochemical abnormalities. It appears to act by decreasing hepatic iron stores, although the precise mechanism is uncertain. 400–500 ml of blood is removed every 1–2 weeks until either a fall in haemoglobin concentration, a fall in plasma ferritin, or a transferrin saturation of less than 15% indicates the beginning of iron deficiency. This usually requires less than 10 venesections. Clinical and biochemical remission follows within a few months in most patients and often lasts for many years without relapse. Alternatively, remission may be induced by administration of chloroquine or hydroxychloroquine. These compounds provoke the release of stored uroporphyrin from the liver, probably by forming water-soluble complexes, and may also deplete hepatic iron stores. Large, antimalarial doses of these drugs produce a severe hepatotoxic reaction in patients with PCT, but low doses (125 mg twice weekly for adults) are well-tolerated and produce remission without any apparent worsening of the liver cell damage that is already present in most patients. In children with PCT, smaller doses are required. The related disorder, hepatoerythropoietic porphyria, in which there is severe hepatic uroporphyrinogen decarboxylase deficiency, does not respond to venesection or to chloroquine.

Management of acute hepatic porphyrias

The treatment of acute attacks of porphyria has been reviewed[2] and will not be described here. There are no specific measures for the treatment of the skin lesions of variegate porphyria and hereditary coproporphyria. In the United Kingdom, the lesions are rarely severe and often remit spontaneously; protective clothing and sunscreen preparations may be helpful.

Since these conditions are inherited as autosomal dominant traits, an important aspect of their management is to initiate family studies to identify latent porphyrics. Such individuals can then be warned to avoid drugs, calorie restriction, alcohol and other factors that are known to precipitate attacks of acute porphyria[2,23].

REFERENCES

1. McColl, K. E. L. and Goldberg, A. (1980). Abnormal porphyrin metabolism in diseases other than porphyria. *Clin. Haematol.*, **9**, 427–51
2. Brodie, M. J. and Goldberg, A. (1980). Acute hepatic porphyrias. *Clin. Haematol.*, **9**, 253–72
3. Doss, M. (1986). Enzymatic deficiencies in acute hepatic porphyrias: porphobilinogen synthase deficiency. *Semin. Dermatol.*, **5**, 161–8

4. Fujita, H., Sassa, S., Toback, A.C. and Kappas, A. (1987). Immunochemical study of uroporphyrinogen decarboxylase in a patient with mild hepatoerythropoietic porphyria. *J. Clin. Invest.*, **79,** 1533–7
5. Murphy, G.M., Hawk, J.L.M., Barrett, D.F., *et al.* (1986). Homozygous variegate porphyria. Two cases in unrelated families. *J. R. Soc. Med.*, **79,** 361–2
6. Desnick, R.J., Ostasiewicz, L., Tischler, P., *et al.* (1985). Acute intermittent porphyria: characterization of a novel mutation in the structural gene for porphobilinogen deaminase. *J. Clin. Invest.*, **76,** 865–74
7. Epstein, J.H., Tuffanelli, D.L. and Epstein, W.L. (1973). Cutaneous changes in the porphyrias – a microscopic study. *Arch. Dermatol.*, **107,** 689–98
8. Magnus, I.A. (1980). Cutaneous porphyrias. *Clin. Haematol.*, **9,** 273–302
9. Poh-Fitzpatrick, M.B. (1982). Pathogenesis and treatment of photocutaneous manifestations of the porphyrias. *Semin. Liver Dis.*, **2,** 164–76
10. Spikes, J.D. (1984). Photobiology of porphyrins. In *Porphyrin Localization and Treatment of Tumors,* pp. 19–39. (New York: Alan R. Liss)
11. Bengtsson, N.O. and Hardell, L. (1986). Porphyrias, porphyrins and hepatocellular cancer. *Br. J. Cancer.*, **54,** 115–17
12. Nordmann, Y. and Deybach, J.C. (1986). Congenital erythropoietic porphyria. *Semin. Dermatol.*, **5,** 106–14
13. Elder, G.H., Urquhart, A.J., Salamanca, R. de E., *et al.* (1985). Immunoreactive uroporphyrinogen decarboxylase in the liver in porphyria cutanea tarda. *Lancet,* **1,** 229–32
14. Cripps, D.J., Peters, H.A., Gocmen, A. and Dogramaci, I. (1984). Porphyria turcica due to hexachlorobenzene: a 20 to 30 year follow-up study on 204 patients. *Br. J. Dermatol.*, **111,** 413–22
15. Grossman, M.E., Bickers, D.R., Poh-Fitzpatrick, M.B., DeLeo, V.A. and Harber, L.C. (1978). Porphyria cutanea tarda: Clinical features and laboratory findings in 40 patients. *Am. J. Med.*, **67,** 277–86
16. Cortes, J., Oliva, H., Paradinas, F.J., *et al.* (1980). The pathology of the liver in porphyria cutanea tarda. *Histopathology,* **4,** 471–85
17. DeLeo, V.A., Poh-Fitzpatrick, M.B., Matthews-Roth, M.M., *et al.* (1976). Erythropoietic protoporphyria: ten years experience. *Am. J. Med.*, **60,** 8–22
18. Bloomer, J.R. (1982). Protoporphyria. *Semin. Liver Dis.*, **2,** 143–53
19. Elder, G.H. (1980). The porphyrias: clinical chemistry, diagnosis and methodology. *Clin. Haematol.*, **9,** 371–98
20. Rimington, C. and Cripps, D.J. (1965). Biochemical and fluorescence microscopy screening tests for erythropoietic protoporphyria. *Lancet,* **1,** 624–6
21. Poh-Fitzpatrick, M.B. (1980). A plasma porphyrin fluorescence marker for variegate porphyria. *Arch. Dermatol.*, **116,** 543–7
22. Harber, L.C. and Bickers, D.R. (1984). Porphyria and pseudoporphyria. *J. Invest. Dermatol.*, **82,** 207–9
23. Bickers, D.R. and Merk, H. (1986). The treatment of porphyrias. *Semin. Dermatol.*, **5,** 186–97
24. Hathum, J. van, Baart de la Faille, H., Van den Berg, J.W.O., *et al.* (1986). Chenodeoxycholic acid therapy in erythrohepatic protoporphyria. *J. Hepatol.*, **3,** 407–12

Index

GPSR Compliance

The European Union's (EU) General Product Safety Regulation (GPSR) is a set of rules that requires consumer products to be safe and our obligations to ensure this.

If you have any concerns about our products, you can contact us on ProductSafety@springernature.com

In case Publisher is established outside the EU, the EU authorized representative is:

Springer Nature Customer Service Center GmbH
Europaplatz 3
69115 Heidelberg, Germany

Batch number: 10607224

Printed by Printforce, the Netherlands